Case Studies of Nursing
Intervention

Case Studies of Nursing Intervention

Department of Nursing Education
University of Kansas Medical Center
Kansas City, Kansas

McGraw-Hill Book Company

A Blakiston Publication

New York St. Louis San Francisco Düsseldorf Johannesburg
Kuala Lumpur London Mexico Montreal New Delhi Panama
Paris São Paulo Singapore Sydney Tokyo Toronto

Case Studies of Nursing Intervention

1234567890 DODO 7987654

Library of Congress Cataloging in Publication Data

Kansas. University. Dept. of Nursing Education.
  Case studies of nursing intervention.

  "A Blakiston publication."
    1. Medicine—Cases, clinical reports, statistics.
2. Nurses and nursing—Cases, clinical reports,
statistics. I. Title. [DNLM: 1. Nursing care—
Case studies. WY100 U78c 1974]
RC66.K36 1974   610.73   73-14753
ISBN 0-07-016425-8

This book was set in Caledonia by Cobb/Dunlop,
    Publisher Services Inc.
The editor was Cathy Dilworth; the designer was
    Cobb/Dunlop; and the production supervisor
    was Judi Frey.
R. R. Donnelley & Sons Company was the printer
    and the binder.

Contents

List of Authors

Martha Underwood Barnard, R.N., B.S.N., M.N.
Assistant Professor and Nurse Clinician, Department of Nursing Education, Department of Human Ecology, University of Kansas Medical Center, Kansas City, Kansas

Sandra Tweed Blades, R.N., B.S.N., M.S.
Assistant Professor, Department of Nursing Education, University of Kansas Medical Center, Kansas City, Kansas

Carolyn Herrington Brose, R.N., B.S.N., M.S.
Director, Department of Nursing Education, William Jewell College, Liberty, Missouri

Judith Troyer Caudle, R.N., B.S.N., M.S.N.
Instructor, Department of Nursing Education, University of Kansas Medical Center, Kansas City, Kansas

Barbara Clancy, R.N., B.S.N., M.S.N.
Assistant Professor, Department of Nursing Education, University of Kansas Medical Center, Kansas City, Kansas

Rita Harris Clifford, R.N., B.S.N., M.S.
Associate Professor, Department of Nursing Education, University of Kansas Medical Center, Kansas City, Kansas

Elaine Darst, R.N., B.S.N., M.S.N.
Psychiatric Nurse, Northeast Kansas Mental Health Center

Lucille D. Gress, R.N., B.S.N., M.A.
Assistant Professor, Department of Nursing Education, University of Kansas Medical Center, Kansas City, Kansas

Sara Hammes, R.N., B.S.N., M.S.N.
Instructor, Department of Nursing Education, University of Kansas Medical Center, Kansas City, Kansas

Rosemary Cannon Kilker, R.N., B.S., M.S.
Associate Professor, Department of Nursing Education, University of Kansas Medical Center, Kansas City, Kansas

Loren O. King, R.N., B.S.N., M.N.
Assistant Professor, Department of Nursing Education, University of Kansas Medical Center, Kansas City, Kansas

Lily Larson, R.N., B.S.N., M.Ed.
Associate Professor, Department of Nursing Education, University of Kansas Medical Center, Kansas City, Kansas

Margaret Shandor Miles, R.N., B.S.N., M.N.
Graduate Student, University of Missouri, Kansas City, Missouri

Margaret R. Peterson, R.N., B.S.N., P.H.N., M.A.
Associate Professor, Department of Nursing Education, University of Kansas Medical Center, Kansas City, Kansas

Jeanne Quesenbury, R.N., B.S., M.N.
Associate Professor, Department of Nursing Education, University of Kansas Medical Center, Kansas City, Kansas

Jeanne R. Schott, R.N., B.S.N., M.S.
Assistant Professor, Department of Nursing Education, University of Kansas Medical Center, Kansas City, Kansas

Margo Lyman Thompson, R.N., B.S.N.
Instructor, Department of Nursing Education, University of Kansas Medical Center, Kansas City, Kansas

Betty L. Wilkerson, R.N., B.S.N., M.A.
Assistant Professor, Department of Nursing Education, University of Kansas Medical Center, Kansas City, Kansas

Lorraine Wolf, R.N., B.S.N., M.A.
Associate Professor, Department of Nursing Education, University of Kansas Medical Center, Kansas City, Kansas

Jean A. Yokes, R.N., B.S.N., M.S.N.
Coordinator, Medical-Surgical Nursing Practice, American Nurses' Association, Kansas City, Missouri

Editor, Case Studies of Nursing Intervention

Marjorie Duffey, R.N., PH.D.
Professor of Nursing and Curriculum Coordinator, Department of Nursing Education, University of Kansas Medical Center, Kansas City, Kansas

Preface

The clinical nursing course in the baccalaureate program for which these case studies were developed focuses on the relationships among nursing, biological, and social science concepts as they relate to complex health problems and promotion of health. Complex health problems are determined by the degree of physical, social, and/or emotional impairment.

Included among the objectives of this clinical course was for the student to develop the ability to evaluate the nursing plan, to plan nursing intervention, and to suggest nursing alternatives. This book of case studies is intended to serve as a basis for discussion in which students and faculty will carry out the evaluative process.

It is our belief, as a faculty, that the nursing student needs such a working model of the essential components of nursing care. The individual case studies were developed by faculty members who had direct personal experience in giving nursing care to these patients.

There were three general criteria used by the faculty to determine which cases should be included in this book: (1) the ages of the individuals should vary from very young children to senior adults; (2) the gravity of the medical problems should vary in stages of acuteness and chronicity; and (3) the health problems represented in the various cases should relate to the prevalence of those health problems in the general population.

Each author was encouraged to use the style of presentation most comfortable for him and the material he was presenting, but in order to be sure that these cases would include the information the faculty felt necessary for their purpose, broad guidelines were established. Each case study would provide information enabling the reader to perceive the interactions among the physical, psychological, and sociological aspects of the particular individual's situation; would require analysis of nursing actions—evaluating the effects of actions taken and stimulating the conceptualization of alternative nursing interventions. To provide some uniformity of format, it was determined that a minimum/maximum number of study questions be set and that pertinent bibliographies be included as suggested readings.

The student is encouraged to familiarize himself with each case study, suggested bibliography, and study guide questions. It is hoped this will serve as a starting point and that the individual student, on her own initiative, will further investigate material not presented in the case studies.

Marjorie Duffey

Case Studies of Nursing Intervention

Andy Sparks
twelve months old

Child Abuse/Acute and Chronic
Martha Underwood Barnard

There are "more deaths attributed to child abuse than are caused by automobile accidents, leukemia, cystic fibrosis, and muscular dystrophy combined."[*] Of these, 50 percent are repeated attacks.[†] These overwhelming facts should make nurses aware of the vital role they have in predicting child abuse as well as in assisting physicians to diagnose child abuse.

The following is a case study to help illustrate child abuse. Andy Sparks, diagnosis: fracture, complete, closed, midshaft femur.

On April 1, 1971, this twelve-month-old white male was admitted to a hospital because the mother had observed that the infant was not moving his right leg. The mother told the doctor that her infant son had caught his leg between the crib bars earlier on April 1. The mother had initially told the emergency room nurse that her infant son had caught his right leg between the railing of his bed and the wall.

(APRIL 1, 1971)

NURSING HISTORY

Patient Profile

This is a twelve-month-old infant who lives in a small white frame home in a rural area outside of Richmond, Kansas, with his mother. His mother is sixteen years old and his father is eighteen years old. Both are in good health and give no history of illness. His father is presently in jail for beating the infant. Both parents have been living together in the home for most of this infant's life. The home has two bedrooms, kitchen, dining area, living room, and indoor bathroom.

[*] Marian Hall, "The Right to Live," *Nursing Outlook*, Vol. 15, August 1967, pp. 56–67.
[†] Ibid., p. 64.

1

Medical History

Chief complaint: "Can't move his right leg."

History of present illness: The patient was brought to the emergency room at 8:03 P.M. today with the complaint of getting his right leg caught in the crib bars. His mother had put him to bed for his nap at 4:05 P.M. She heard him crying at 6:00 P.M., at which time she found him caught. The right thigh was red and swollen; he did not move his leg much and did not like anyone to touch it.

Past Medical History

Antenatal history: Gravidal Para 1, living children 1. Born at this hospital, this child is a product of an unwanted pregnancy. He weighed 6.7 kg at birth. Apgars were 7 and 9, respectively. The mother stated that she started having antenatal checkups at this medical center at four months. She took iron, calcium, and vitamins during her pregnancy and states that she took no other drugs. She gives no history of drinking any alcohol during her pregnancy, smoked a pack of cigarettes each day, and occasionally drank coffee. She denies having any depression during any part of her pregnancy. She gained 11.25 kg during pregnancy and had no headaches or hypertension during this time. The mother states that because of an "inadequate pelvis" a cesarean section was performed. Mother and infant went home together four days after delivery. The mother has an intrauterine device at present.

Infant Past Medical History

Six-week DPT was given; no other immunizations were given. The mother states the infant "cried a lot during his younger months and spit up a lot." She gives a history of diarrhea at three months and a "bad diaper rash around six months." The infant was not seen for these problems by a physician or a nurse.

Social and Family History

Father.
Eighteen-year-old Caucasian
Living and apparently in good physical health
Grade school education
Two years of high school; worked as automobile mechanic, gas station attendant, and farm worker since dropping out of high school three years previous to March 1971. Mother and father both living. Parents were separated most of the eighteen-year-old's life.
Social habits: Smokes one pack of cigarettes a day, occasionally smokes marijuana, drinks beer only.

Mother.
Sixteen-year-old Caucasian
Living and apparently well
Not married
Reared by her maternal grandparents her entire life
Occasionally lived with an aunt during summers
Completed grade school
Completed one semester of high school
Social habits: Drinks beer and hard liquor, smokes cigarettes occasionally, denies any use of drugs.

Maternal grandfather.
Living and well

Maternal grandmother.
Living, had cancer of the uterus. Total hysterectomy performed three years ago. Under medical care.

Paternal grandmother.
Living and has arthritis of both hands. Under medical care.

Paternal grandfather.
Living and has a duodenal ulcer. Under medical care.

The family is supported by welfare at $300 a month. On being asked what her biggest problem was with Andy, the mother stated, "his temper. If we tell him no, he will start to scream." I asked what she did then and she said, "I ignore him." Then she pulled out a *Better Homes and Gardens Book for Infant Care.* "I read in here to put him in his room and ignore him. His father is better than I am. He puts him in his room, tells him to be quiet, and leaves him there. Andy minds his daddy." I then asked her what else they do to discipline the child. "Tell him 'NO, NO,' or if he's doing something he shouldn't, I'll slap his hands."

Eating habits. Skim milk. Two 8-oz bottles between his three meals. Sometimes he will cup feed with help during his meals. Not quite sure of total amount of milk he drinks per day. Eats table foods—meat and vegetables. Has not been given fruits.
Bowel habits. Soft stools. Has three or more per day. No history of constipation or diarrhea.
Voiding. Normal. Smell not strong. Does not appear heavily concentrated.
Sleep habits. Occasional nap during the day. Sleeps through the night. No history of nightmares.

Growth/development patterns. Weight 7.65 kg, Height 29 in., Head Circumference 19 in. Smiles. Three-word vocabulary: Mama, Dada, and shut up. Gurgles. Sits up without support; can get into sitting position on his own. Cannot crawl. When placed on his abdomen, he pulls with his hands, drags right leg, and flexes his left leg. By doing this, he pushes off on his left leg, scooting himself around on his abdomen. If placed on his feet, he stands on both feet, again extending his right leg, flexing and kneeling on his left leg. He then pulls himself to a standing position and puts his weight on both feet. When given support while in a standing position, he moves both legs in a walking motion. Very cooperative during examination. Cried slightly once. Showed no resistance throughout examination. Grasps reflex strong on both sides. Follows bright colors and flashlight.

Physical Examination

Head. Circumference 19 in.; anterior and posterior fontanel closed; no cuts, scratches, burns, or bruises. Hair is matted with old milk.

Eyes. Pupils equal and reactive to light, corneal light reflex equal, scelera clear, conjunctiva slightly pale. Bilateral red reflex.

Ears. Dirt in outer auricle, old milk behind both ears, small amount of cerumen in right ear and large amount in left ear. Bilateral light reflex of both tympanic membranes. No cuts, scratches, or bruises.

Nose. No drainage; both nares patent.

Throat. Normal.

Mouth. No signs of dehydration; nine teeth; cutting one tooth now; drooling.

Neck. No enlarged nodes. Moves head with ease.

Chest. Respiration 30 and regular. Clear upon auscultation. Did not appear sore on any part of the thorax. No cuts, burns, or bruises.

Heart. No murmur; regular, 110 rate.

Abdomen. Can feel slight tip of liver 1½ cm below middle right costal margin. No masses. Did not appear sore or tender while being palpated. No cuts, burns, or bruises.

Hips. 180° rotation.

Genitalia. Normal male; circumcized penis; both testes descended.

Buttocks, anus. Slight diaper rash.

Torso. Normal; no scoliosis. No cuts, burns, or bruises. Appears slightly thin.

Skin. Slight diaper rash. Two bruises over left malar eminence. Two blisters those oppose each other when elbow is flexed on the forearm.

CNS. No moro; good grasp, no head lag. Bilateral Babinski. Normal deep tendon reflexes.

Extremities. Flexes and extends all four extremities while on his back. Hands, normal creases and palms pink. Feet clean, pink, and no clubbing.

PROBLEMS

1. Limited movement of the right leg
2. Developmental lag in the gross motor area
3. Bruises and blisters of unknown origin
4. Failure to gain weight
5. Inadequate diet according to history
6. Questionable social history

PLAN

1.01 Do Denver Developmental Screening Test today by nurse clinician
1.02 Refer to Neurology for neurological developmental assessment
1.03 Refer to Jody Barnes, R.N., P.N.C., for developmental stimulation evaluation
1.04 Refer to Marge Brown, R.N., for play evaluation
2.01 Refer to orthopedic service or orthopedic workup
2.02 Obtain skeletal x rays
3.01 Refer to child protective team to rule out child abuse
3.02 Admit to 2 West
4.01 Refer to Endocrine Clinic for weight evaluation
5.01 Refer to department of dietetics for diet evaluation
5.02 Evaluate family diet
6.01 Make home referral to Public Health Department
6.02 Refer to social service
6.03 Contact family's welfare office

Martha U. Barnard, R.N.
Pediatric Nurse Clinician

ORTHOPEDIC PHYSICAL EXAMINATION AND TREATMENT

Physical Exam

Temperature. 37.2°.; pulse 130; respiration 36

H.E.E.N.T. Fontanelles—posterior closed, anterior ½ by 1 cm soft and appears normal. Pupils equal and reactive to light. Throat clear. Tympanic membrane clear.

Neck. Supple without adenopathy

Chest. Clear to auscultation

Heart. Regular sinus rhythms; no murmurs

Abdomen. No masses or organomegaly

Extremities. Within normal limits except tender and swollen; slightly firm right thigh with the knee at 100° flexion

Skin. Has bruises 2 to 3 days old (estimated) over the left malar eminence and small blisters that oppose one another when the elbow is flexed on the arm and forearm

Neurological Exam

Bilateral Babinskies; good strong root and suck reflex.

Laboratory.

UA: pH 615; Sp. gr. 1.023
CBC: Hg 12.8; Hct. 40; W.B.C. 13,630
PKU: Negative
Skeletal x rays: No abnormalities except for the following: x ray of the right femur showed a transverse complete fracture of the right femoral midshaft.

Diagnosis. fracture, complete, midshaft femur

Operation and procedures. application of body spica plaster

FIRST ADMISSION HOSPITAL COURSE

The patient was given 12.5 mg of Demerol and 7.0 mg of Phenergan intramuscularly in the emergency room and placed on the infant fracture table and was placed in a body spica incorporating both legs to the toes. The patient did well in the hospital and was discharged April 4. He was asked to return to the Orthopedic Clinic on April 12.

Referrals

V.N.A. "To see about proper well baby care."

Medical Orders

First admission order sheet:
April 1, 1971

1. Admit to 3 L
2. Temperature q. 6 h.; vital signs B.I.D.
3. Check circulation and motion of both feet q. 2 h.
4. C.B.C. in A.M.
5. U.A. in A.M.
6. Elevate feet 4 to 6 in. tonight
7. Ice pack to right thigh
8. Regular diet for age
9. Benadryl, 10 mg—elixir q. 4 h. p.r.n. for restlessness

April 4, 1971

1. Discharge
2. Return to Orthopedic Clinic on April 12

Visiting Nurse's Association Report

A public health nurse went to make a home visit concerning this infant. The mother and infant had moved from the address given in the referral and had left no forwarding address.

FLOOR NURSE'S NOTES—FIRST ADMISSION

April 1, 1971   12 midnight
A twelve-month-old male admitted per cart from E.R. In spica cast CC "Fx femur (R)." Bagged for U.A. Has voided and had one stool. Legs elevated; ice bags to the Fx. Toes cool to touch but has good capillary return. Moves toes easily with stimulation. Dr. Glenn here, also both parents.

2 A.M.
Fussy. Benadryl Elixer 10 mg given.

6–7 A.M.
Turned on abdomen with legs elevated. Ice bag to thigh. Toes remain cool, but he has good capillary return; moves them easily after stimulation. A fairly good night.

April 2, 1971   7–8 A.M.
Parents here to feed in A.M. Ice pack to R femur. Legs elevated. Parents left.

11–3 P.M.
Elevation and ice pack dc'd. Ate well. Placed in wagon and out in halls for stimulation. Toes cool but blanch, good motion.

3–11 P.M.
Taking purees well and formula poor. Toes warm and good color. Able to move toes. No temp. elevation.

April 3, 1971   12–7 A.M.
Sleep. Urine collected to direct drainage. Supine position; turned x2. Sweet milk taken.

8 A.M.
Ate breakfast well. Toes blanch well. Fussy except when held. No temp. elevation. Turned to abdomen. Fussy for a while, then asleep.

1 P.M.
Ate well for lunch. Doesn't take fluids very well. Circulation remains good in toes.

3–11 P.M.
Crying most of evening. Ate purees well, took fluids poorly. Circulation appears good.

April 4, 1971   12–7 A.M.
Sleeping, turned. Circulation, etc., good.

1:30 P.M.
Dismissed to parent with return appointment for x ray.

SECOND ADMISSION

The patient was not brought back to the clinic until April 17. At this time it was decided to admit the patient to the pediatrics unit.

Doctor's Order on Second Admission
April 17, 1971

1. Admit to 3 L Ortho
2. Dx old fracture of the right femur
3. V.S. q.d.; temp. q. 6 h. rectally
4. C.B.C. by finger stick in A.M.
5. U.A. today
6. Cast care
7. Two-pound Bryant's traction on right side
8. Regular diet for age
9. Nebulizer to bedside at all times
10. Benadryl 12.5 mg P.O. q. 6 h. for restlessness
11. Actifed ¼ tsp. t.i.d.

After admission the infant was taken out of his spica cast and placed in Bryant's traction with 90° hip flexion. The patient had been kept in a croupette during his entire hospitalization due to expiratory croup. This croup improved during the six days he was in the hospital.

On April 21, 1971, Andy was taken out of his Bryant's traction and placed in a spica cast.

On the day of discharge Andy's mother was advised to obtain a vaporizer to use on the child at all times and to notify the physician if the croup became more severe. She was also instructed on pedaling the cast and how to keep the cast clean.

The infant was finally discharged on April 24, 1971.

FLOOR NURSE'S NOTES—SECOND ADMISSION

April 17, 1971   3:30 P.M.
A twelve-month-old male admitted per w/c from clinic to have casted leg placed in traction. Accompanied by mother. U.A. not immediately obtained. Patient bagged.

5 P.M.
Dr. Glenn here to set up traction.

6 P.M.
Eating poorly. Sucking bottle of milk.

8:30 P.M.
Croupette set up in place of vaporizer for croup.

11 P.M.
Bagged to dependent drainage to keep cast dry. No weight taken.

April 18, 1971   12–6 A.M.
Slept well. Remains in croupette.

7–11 A.M.
Ate good breakfast. Out of croupette, appears to be tolerating well. Remains in traction.

12–3 P.M.
Sleeping between feeding.

3–11 P.M.
Leg remains in traction. Toes warm and good color. Out of croupette. Croupy cough several times. Portable chest x ray done. Patient to x ray per bed and back to floor. No temp. elevation. Appetite fairly good.

April 19, 1971   11–1 A.M.
Sleeping. Taking fluids well. Urinary collection bag reapplied. Remains in traction.

7–3 P.M.
Partial sponge bath. Appetite fair. Playful, moving toes well.

3–11 P.M.
Appetite fair. No temp. elevation. Circulation in toes good. Patient's temp. 36.9°C. at 7 P.M. Patient irritable and crying a lot.

12–6 A.M.
Appears to be sleeping.

April 20, 1971   7–11 A.M.
Patient's appetite good, takes fluids slowly. B.M. 7:45 A.M. Changed urine bag 10 A.M. Breathing occasionally raspy and labored. Choked x3 while eating. Coughs and expectorates x1, mostly food. Cough and swallow most of time. Sensation in toes. Color pink. Moves toes constantly. Very active.

11–1 P.M.
Sleeping.

3–11 P.M.
Toes warm and circulation good. Vomited x2, small amounts. Ate well for supper, taking fluids poorly.

April 21, 1971   12–7 A.M.
Sleeping, circulation in toes good.

7–8 A.M.
Had large stool, brown. Sponge bath with complete linen change.

3–11 P.M.
Good evening. Took purees well. Fluids poorly. Voiding one brown soft stool.

April 22, 1971   12–7 A.M.
Slept. Circulation good.

7–9 A.M.
Patient had A.M. care. Ate fairly well at breakfast. Circulation in toes appears good. Wiggling of toes noted also. B.P. unable to be obtained.

9–1:30 P.M.
T.P.R. at 1 = 37°C 124, 24. Circulation appears good with repeated wiggling of toes. Intake of 540. Bagged urine app. stool x2.

3–11 P.M.
Toes warm and good color. Wiggling toes on his own. Had croupy cough while eating supper. Taking formula poorly.

April 23, 1971   12–7 A.M.
Sleeping.

7–10 A.M.
Appetite good, drank O.J. for breakfast. Had bath, voiding well. To E.R.

1 P.M.
Back from E.R., circulation in toes good. Ate lunch; no temp.

5:25 P.M.
Vomited x5. Dr. Glenn called: Put back into croupette. Had a hard-formed stool, moderate amount. Sounds croupy. Vomited again small amount. Toes warm and good color. Able to wiggle toes.

April 24, 1971   12–7 A.M.
Sleeping in croupette. Circulation good.

7–2 P.M.
Coughed very little. Ate well. Voiding well. Taking fluids well. Moderate, soft brown stool.

2 P.M.
Dismissed to parents after Dr. Glenn talked to mother on phone. Parents instructed on pedaling cast when dry and keeping plaster in place, to keep cast from getting wet.

SUMMARY OF SOCIAL SERVICE INTERVENTION

The pediatric nurse clinician was contacted because of the concern of the Richmond welfare workers about this child on April 1. Neighbors had reported to the local welfare agency that the eighteen-year-old father had been seen "whipping" him on several occasions. Three times the neighbors reported that there was no apparent reason for punishing the infant. Twice the father punished the infant because he was going "to show the mother she better move into the same home with him if she expected him to act like a nice father."

The child was examined and referred to the orthopedic medical staff, where the diagnosis of a fractured femur was made. The child has been followed for approximately one month and one week. During that time he was admitted to the hospital two times, April 1 and April 17.

During both hospitalizations physicians did not feel that there was sufficient medical evidence to validate a diagnosis of child abuse or suspected child abuse.

On April 24, 1971, the day of discharge, the Richmond welfare workers resumed their investigation of this case. After one week they got a court order to temporarily remove the child from the custody of his mother. At this time the mother told juvenile authorities that the child's father had beaten the infant on several occasions, one of which resulted in an injury to the infant's right leg. Juvenile authorities reported this to local law enforcement agents. The father was then arrested. He is now in the custody of the law and awaiting trial.

On May 3, 1971, the infant was placed back in the home with his mother after being in a foster home for three days. The mother and infant were placed on welfare funds. The mother and infant have not been seen by relatives or any law enforcement agents for two weeks. The hospital also reported that the mother did not bring the infant in for two clinic appointments after the second admission.

STUDY GUIDE

1. What baseline data should the nurse collect for her initial nursing assessment on any child admitted to the pediatrics unit?
2. Of these baseline data what would be considered the most significant in predicting possible child abuse?
3. What characteristics of this case study would make you suspect classic child abuse?
4. What additional information should have been collected by physicians, nurses, and welfare workers?
5. What referrals should have been made by individuals on the health team
    a. to report to
    b. for consultation.
6. Who is responsible for reporting suspected child abuse in your state?
7. What would be some tactful methods of obtaining information from parents or a guardian of a suspected abused child or an abused child?
8. What things would be important to identify about growth and developmental patterns of any child with suspected child abuse?
9. What things would be important to identify about growth and developmental patterns of this infant?
    a. What is the most common cause of failure to gain weight in children?
10. What physical findings would be important for the nurse to observe on any children with the diagnosis of suspected child abuse?
11. What interaction patterns of children and their parents should be observed?
12. What social characteristics in this study would make you suspect child abuse?
13. Did anything occur during the mother's pregnancy that would make you suspect a possibility of child abuse?
14. Criticize the nurses' notes.
    a. What additional information is needed in these nurses' notes?
    b. What information could have been eliminated?

15. Criticize the medical physical examination. What additional information should be included?
16. Are the laboratory values within normal limits during both admissions?
17. What reactions should the nurse look for in relation to the drugs given during both hospitalizations?
18. On the first admission what type of observations should the nurse have been making in relation to the infant's cast?
19. What should the mother be taught about this infant's cast?
20. Do you think the vital signs were taken often enough? What would be the most significant vital signs with this patient?
21. Why was the ice pack being placed on the right thigh?
22. What is a spica cast?
23. What is the purpose of a spica cast?
24. What is the difference between skin and skeletal traction?
25. What type of traction is Bryant's traction? What is the purpose of Bryant's traction?
26. How can the nurse assess this infant's respiratory status?
27. What early signs and symptoms might indicate respiratory distress?
28. How should you assess older children's respiratory status?
29. What observations might indicate impending skin breakdown?
30. Why might a respiratory infection occur in patients in traction or in spica casts?
31. What nursing action should be included in the care for this infant to prevent decubiti?
32. What nursing care plans would be important for *this* infant?
33. What is a regular diet for a child of this age?
34. Why would it be important to give smaller amounts during each feeding?
35. Make out a home referral for a community nurse. Include your nursing goals for a follow-up visit.
36. Design a nursing assessment tool to be used by a community health nurse on a home visit. Include
    a. environment
    b. social history
    c. family history
    d. physical assessment of children in the home.
37. Compare the content of the nursing history with the nurse's notes.

SELECTED READINGS

Betty S. Bergeson and Elise E. Krug, in consultation with Andres Goth, *Pharmacology in Nursing,* C. V. Mosby, St. Louis, 1969.
T. Berry Brazelton, *Infants and Mothers—Differences in Development,* Dell, New York, 1969.

Debra Hymovich and Martha U. Barnard, *Family Health Care*, McGraw-Hill, New York, 1973, pp. 365–376.

R. S. Illingworth, *Common Symptoms of Disease in Children*, Blackwell Scientific Publications, Oxford, 1971, pp. 1–20.

C. Henry Kempe and Ray E. Helfer, *Helping the Battered Child and His Family*, J. B. Lippincott, Philadelphia, 1972.

Avice Kerr, "Nurses' Notes, Making Them More Meaningful," *Nursing*, vol. 2, no. 9, September 1972, p. 6.

Carroll Larson and Marjorie Gould, *Calderwood's Orthopedic Nursing*, C. V. Mosby, St. Louis, 1965, pp. 61–113.

Dorothy R. Marlow, *Textbook of Pediatric Nursing*, W. B. Saunders, Philadelphia, 1968.

Waldo Emerson Nelson, *Textbook of Pediatrics*, W. B. Saunders, Philadelphia, 1969, pp. 127–160.

Madeline Petrillo and Sirgay Sanger, *Emotional Care of Hospitalized Children*, J. B. Lippincott, Philadelphia, 1972, pp. 19–122.

Fairfax T. Proudfit and Corine H. Robinson, *Normal and Therapeutic Nutrition*, Macmillan, New York, 1967.

Jeanne Holman Quesenbury and Pamela Lembright, "Observations and Care for Patients with Head Injuries," *The Nursing Clinics of North America*, vol. 4, no. 2, June 1969, pp. 237–247.

Jane Secor, *Patient Care in Respiratory Problems*, W. B. Saunders, Philadelphia, 1969, pp. 77–90.

Diane Rose
two-and-one-half years old

Lye Ingestion/Acute
Margaret Shandor Miles

This study of Diane should help the student apply the steps in the nursing process to the care of a hospitalized toddler. The steps that are illustrated include data collection, developing a nursing problem list and plan of care, nursing intervention as illustrated by process recordings, and evaluation.

The sources of data used in this study of Diane include the medical history and medical orders, a discussion with the nursing staff about Diane's response to hospitalization and procedures, a nursing history collected from Diane's parents, and an assessment of Diane by the author.

From the data collected, a tentative nursing diagnosis, or problem list, was developed. For each problem a nursing plan is outlined that is aimed at helping Diane cope with the problems created by the sudden illness and hospitalization. The problems listed and the nursing plans overlap and cannot be considered separate, isolated entities. The list helps to illustrate sources of stress for a hospitalized toddler.

An attempt is made to illustrate the author's nursing intervention with Diane by use of process recordings and evaluative comments. The intervention with her parents is not included in this study. For further information about the care of Diane and her parents, see the articles in the bibliography by Miles and Barnes.

At the end of the study, evaluation of the nursing intervention, based upon the problem list and plan of care, is presented.

DATA COLLECTION

Medical History and Orders

Diane is a two-and-one-half-year-old girl who was hospitalized in a 290-bed metropolitan children's hospital for lye ingestion. Diane drank some of the lye and had given some to her nine-month-old sister, Jean.

The children were admitted to this hospital after preliminary treatment

15

at a community hospital. Jean did not swallow the lye, but suffered severe burns of the chin and lips. She was hospitalized in the infant unit and was discharged after two and one-half weeks.

Diane's diagnosis on admission was burns of the mouth, pharynx, tongue, palate, and uvula. There were also slight burns on the neck and between two fingers of her right hand. Her mouth and throat were swollen and painful. She experienced much difficulty swallowing, and excess amounts of saliva drooled from her mouth, necessitating frequent suctioning. For several days fluids were given only by intravenous feedings; gradually fluids by mouth were permitted, but swallowing was painful and difficult. Besides the oral suctioning, some of the treatment and diagnostic measures had included esophagoscopy and laryngoscopy under anesthesia, frequent examinations of the mouth, application of mineral oil and antibiotic ointment to lesions of the mouth and lips, extraction of several teeth, and oral dilatation of the esophagus with a bougie to prevent a stricture from developing.

The medical orders at the time this study began (ninth hospital day) included

1. urge fluids
2. full liquid diet as tolerated
3. mineral oil q.i.d.
4. observe for signs of esophageal rupture
5. T.P.R. q. 4 h.
6. out of bed as desired
7. antibiotic ointment to lips—finger wound q.i.d.

NURSING HISTORY

Pertinent Prior Health Care Experiences

The child has never been in a hospital before; she has had normal childhood infections such as colds, diarrhea, etc.

Patient's Understanding of This Illness

As Diane is only two-and-one-half years old, no one seems to know what she understands about the hospitalization and procedures. Her parents, not knowing what to tell her, or how, have not explained anything.

Parents' Understanding of This Illness

Mr. and Mrs. Rose have a limited understanding of the burns and the current treatment. They have many questions and do not seem to understand the long-term implications of the esophageal burn.

Events Leading to Present Hospitalization

On the evening of the accident which hospitalized Diane and her sister, Jean, nine months old, the children were in their beds, but remained awake to await their father's return from the evening shift. While their mother was in the basement for a brief period, Diane went into the kitchen, climbed onto the sink, and obtained a can of lye stored behind the curtain on the window ledge. She returned to the bedroom, ingested a quantity of the caustic substance, and also fed some to Jean. Mrs. Rose discovered the accident when both children began to cry hysterically.

Preparation for Hospitalization

There was none. The children were rushed to the community hospital and then to the medical center, where they were admitted amidst great confusion.

Parents' Expectations

The parents were very concerned about Diane's withdrawn and depressed behavior. They do not know what to expect and do not know how to relate to her. This seems to be their main concern.

Family Data

Mrs. Rose is a twenty-three-year-old housewife. She appears rather timid, but is able to ask appropriate questions.

Mr. Rose is a twenty-six-year-old electrician. He appears to be concerned about the children and supportive of his wife.

Jean is the nine-month-old sister. She is hospitalized in the infant unit for severe burns of the chin and lips.

Family lives 59 miles from the medical center in a small rural community. The family enjoys doing many activities together.

Financial situation. They have hospitalization. Their income is moderate.

Significant Data about Diane

Appearance. Diane is a sad, depressed, frightened child who sits in the corner of her bed and does not relate to anyone. Saliva drools from the corner of her mouth.

Mother's description of Diane. She is usually a very active, happy child who relates well to people. The parents are concerned about the abrupt change in her behavior.

Developmental history. Diane could stand while holding onto furniture and could sit alone at five months; was walking by seven and one-half months while holding onto furniture; walked alone at twelve months; could feed herself at an early age. By one and one-half years she could mimic any sentence she heard and she started speaking in sentences.

Rest and sleep. At home she sleeps in the same room with Jean, and usually goes to bed quite late, as they stay up for their dad's return from work; she takes a long afternoon nap. Diane is sleeping very poorly in the hospital. She appears afraid to sleep.

Elimination. Diane was toilet-trained during the day, but has now lost control and refuses to use the potty. There is no constipation or other problems at home.

Nutrition. Diane usually has a good appetite. She dislikes few foods. The family usually has a light breakfast, large lunch with dad before going to work, a light supper. No allergies.

Play and activities. Diane is an active child, enjoys outdoor play and dolls, plays well with her sister, has several friends her own age whom she enjoys.

Independence/dependence. She is a very independent child, and likes to dress, feed, and bathe herself. She is close to her parents and depends on them in time of stress.

Temperament. Diane has a temper at times and communicates her anger by screaming and stamping her feet. She does not become angry very often, but reacts when asked to do something or when Jean gets into her tops. She is sensitive when reprimanded and will go to her room and hide.

Interpersonal relationship/communication patterns. Diane is able to talk and can verbally communicate most desires. Some of her pronunciation of words is hard for outsiders to understand. She comprehends what she has been told. She relates well to people, but is shy with strangers.

Skin. Burns are obvious on her lips and right hand. Her chin is red and irritated from drooling mucous, and her skin appears pale and dry.

Respiration. Normal.

Circulation. Normal.

Senses. She had no prior difficulty speaking, but has difficulty now because of the burn and resultant edema and saliva.

Nursing Staff Assessment

The nursing staff reported that Diane was very depressed and withdrawn and would not cooperate with treatments or fluid intake. She refused to eat and drink and refused her medications. She would not go to the playroom or play with any of her toys.

PROBLEM LIST
AND NURSING CARE PLAN

PROBLEM: *Separation Anxiety*

Diane has difficulty coping with the sudden, unexplained separation from her mother, father, sister, and home.°

Plan: To help Diane cope with this abrupt and fearful separation from her mother.

1. To develop a trust relationship with Diane
2. To help her re-establish emotional ties with her parents
3. To help her begin to trust medical personnel
4. To help her understand why she is in the hospital.

PROBLEM: *Body Integrity Fears*

She is frightened by the strange, hospital environment and by the painful things done to her, particularly to her mouth, which is a vulnerable area.

Plan: To help Diane deal with fears about her body integrity.

1. To help her understand body changes secondary to the accident (burns and adhesions of the mouth, hand, esophagus, etc.)
2. To help her understand the treatment measures.

PROBLEM: *Loss of Autonomy*

The striving for autonomy and independence, which has just begun for Diane, is lost by the stresses and the environment itself.

Plan: To assist Diane in regaining and maintaining a sense of autonomy.

1. To allow her control of situations as much as possible (decision making)
2. To respect her attempts at being independent
3. To assist her in regaining control of bladder and bowel.

PROBLEM: *Use of Withdrawal as a Way of Coping with Anger, Fear, and Lack of Trust*

Withdrawal can be a protective device, but it also deprives her of other effective avenues of coping with anxiety such as activity, play, and motion.

° Rooming in was very limited at this hospital but would be strongly recommended for a toddler like Diane.

Plan: To help Diane find other outlets for her feelings and other ways of coping with the stresses of this hospitalization.
1. To help her express feelings of anger and fear about the many things being done to her
2. To provide play opportunities through which she can master and express these feelings.

PROBLEM: *Poor Nutritional State*

The poor intake of food and fluids is caused by four factors: (1) the burns make eating painful; (2) refusing to eat is one activity she can control; (3) fear, withdrawal, and depression decrease the appetite; (4) unfamiliar surroundings and food.

Plan: To assist Diane in accepting adequate intake of food and fluids necessary to promote healing and to increase energy.
1. To allow her to have some control of the feeding situation and at the same time to set limits; i.e., "You can drink this when you want to do so, but we cannot read this book until you have finished it."
2. To provide a full liquid diet high in protein
3. To provide small frequent feedings in attractive containers
4. To make a game out of feedings.

PROBLEM: *Burned Esophagus*

Burns of the tissue and the muscle of the esophagus could cause weakening of the wall, leading to collapse or rupture following dilatation; edema and swelling associated with the burn could cause a stricture; scar tissue could form during healing, causing a stricture.

Plan: To look for signs and symptoms of stricture or rupture of the esophagus.
1. To look for symptoms of choking, coughing after eating, or difficulty in swallowing
2. To look for symptoms of dyspnea, cyanosis, or fatigue
3. To keep suction apparatus at bedside.

PROBLEM: *Infected Burn on Lips*

Plan: To promote healing of the wounds and prevention of infection.
1. To provide adequate nutrition, particularly protein intake
2. To apply antibiotic ointment to wound
3. To clean area, especially after meals.

PROBLEM: *Exhaustion*

Exhaustion is caused by fear of sleeping in this strange environment.

Plan: To promote rest and sleep.

1. The first three problems are related to this lack of sleep; working on them will help her sleep better.
2. Provide a rest period in the afternoon when no one is to disturb her.
3. Stay with her during nap periods on the first few days.
4. Remind her at night when she is going to be alone that her parents love her and will return in the morning, or whenever they will be coming.

PROBLEM: *Anxious and Depressed Parents*

Some of Diane's fears and anxieties could be related to parental attitudes.

Plan: To assist Diane's parents in coping with this sudden hospitalization of their only two children.

1. To listen to their concerns about Diane's and Jean's physical conditions
2. To listen to their expressions of grief about the accident
3. To listen to their concerns about Diane's behavior and to help them understand why Diane is acting as she is
4. To help them understand how they can best help their children during this crisis
5. To answer their questions about the physical problem and treatment measures
6. To help them formulate questions to ask the doctor
7. To help them understand the personnel, policies, and physical plant of this huge medical center.

NURSING INTERVENTION

Initial contact with Diane was made on the ninth day after her hospital admission. The original study covered a period of eighteen months and included two hospitalizations, many outpatient visits for esophageal dilatations, and several home visits. The nursing intervention illustrated in these process recordings, however, focuses on only the first four days of the author's contact with Diane. The recordings for each day represent only part of the interactions that occurred, as the author spent three to four hours a day with Diane and her parents. Comments are made along with the process recordings to evaluate the nursing process and Diane's reactions.

PROCESS RECORDINGS	COMMENTS

Day One (ninth day after admission)

When the nurse first entered the room, Diane looked at her briefly and then stared into space blankly. The nurse put the side rail down and Diane continued to ignore her. The sun seemed to be shining in Diane's eyes so the nurse asked if she wanted the blind pulled down and proceeded to pull it down. She immediately mumbled some words and nodded her head, obviously irritated. "Do you want the blind up?" the nurse asked. Again Diane mumbled and nodded "yes."

Diane expresses her autonomy and the nurse allows her to control by following her decision.

After pulling the blind up, the nurse asked if Diane would like to read a story. No response. "Would you like to read this story," the nurse said as she picked up a book. Diane reluctantly nodded "yes." As the nurse read, Diane remained silent, indicated little response, but stared intently at the nurse. When the nurse offered to read another book, Diane immediately said, "I'm sleepy. You go away." Ignoring her plea, the nurse said, "Would you like to paint." She again mumbled, "Go away," as she began to fuss and cry. "Well, I'll come back later and we can play or read," the nurse said when she left the room.

Rejection. The nurse wanted Diane to know that she was truly interested in her, despite Diane's rejection behavior toward her.

Rejection is hard to take.

When the nurse returned to the room, a volunteer was sitting beside her bed and Diane seemed to accept her presence. She immediately told the nurse to go away. The volunteer left and the nurse produced a story about the "Red Caboose." While reading the story, a little boy came into the room to listen and demanded the nurse's attention. When the nurse turned to him momentarily to answer a question, Diane seemed annoyed.

The volunteer did not have a white uniform on and was not trying to establish a relationship. Rejection again.

A sign of a relationship.

Diane remained more interested in this story, which is about a caboose who strays away from where he was supposed to be, is bad, and then conforms to be accepted again by his elders.

Did Diane identify with the Red Caboose?

The supper tray of full liquids came and Diane refused it. All of the nurse's urging and encouragement did not work. She remained firm about not eating. A milk shake was offered and she agreed to drinking it. When it arrived, however, she refused. "I'll put it here on the table and you can drink it when you are ready. Diane needs to drink to help her get better." After a few minutes, she reached over and drank most of it.

Expressing her independence.

The nurse allowed her to have control over the feeding situation. Interpreting to her the importance of food.

Throughout the time that the nurse was with her, Diane repeatedly called, "My mommy. Where is my mommy. I want my mommy." Knowing that her parents would be visiting at any time, the nurse reassured Diane that they

Constantly reinforcing

PROCESS RECORDINGS *(continued)*	COMMENTS *(continued)*

loved her very much and would be coming to visit her very soon. When her mother arrived, Diane immediately reached for her and sobbed.

and reminding Diane of her parents' love so she won't feel abandoned and unloved.

Day Two (tenth hospital day)

Diane was lying in bed with the same blank stare on her face when the nurse arrived. She became very upset and cried, "Go away. I'm sleepy." The nurse greeted her calmly and sat beside her bed. She put a puppet on her hand. Diane's eyes brightened and she looked at the puppet intently. The puppet began talking: "Diane is a sick girl. She has a sore mouth but it is getting better. She misses her mommy and daddy. She doesn't like the hospital. She doesn't like the things the doctors and nurses must do to her. But she will go home soon. She is getting better and will go home soon." She listened intently and then began to cry, "My mommy. Mommy come back. Mommy come back." The nurse reassured Diane that mommy would come back and that she had a nice mommy who loved her very much and who would take her home soon. This time Diane chanted, "Go away. Go away." Again the nurse said that she would leave, but would return in a few minutes.

Rejection again. Desire to withdraw.
Attempting to relate to Diane through a toy rather than directly, which was too threatening. The nurse is trying to let Diane know that she understands how she feels.

A reminder of her acute need for her mother.

A toddler's rejection can be hard to take.

When the nurse returned, Diane was again staring into space with the same sad, depressed expression. The nurse asked if she would like to visit her sister. Diane stared intently with sorrowful yet happy eyes and nodded "yes." "My sister. My sister," she whispered as they rode down the hall to the elevator. "Your sister has a sore mouth, but it is getting better. She is getting better." Diane was very timid and quiet as she looked at her sister's face intently. The nurse continued to reassure her that Jean was getting better. Soon Diane backed away and said, "Wan' go to room. Wan' go to sleep."

The nurse thought that Diane probably missed her sister, was puzzled by their separation, and was worried about Jean.

Looking at Jean's wounds was too threatening. Need to escape.

Diane immediately climbed into bed upon returning to her room. "Me wan' sleep. Go away." The nurse offered various fluids, reminding her that she needed food to make her well. "Milk shake. Milk shake." When the nurse returned with the shake, Diane didn't want it, so the nurse again placed it on the stand. Diane drank it when she was ready. "Wan' sleep. Go away." The nurse responded, "You sleep, Diane, and I'll sit beside your bed."

Expressed her autonomy.

An attempt to help her feel safe enough to really sleep.

When she awoke from her nap, she asked the nurse to read her a story. After the story, the nurse drew a pic-

A sign of acceptance.

PROCESS RECORDINGS (continued)	COMMENTS (continued)

ture of a little girl and a hospital bed. Then the nurse told Diane a story about a little girl who had a sore mouth and who was very sad and frightened because she must be in the hospital when she wanted to go home. The little girl didn't like the things the doctors and nurses were doing to her. Diane listened quietly. The nurse continued the story saying that the little girl must have these things done to her because they will make her better; when she is better she can go home.

Trying to help her understand why she was in the hospital undergoing painful treatments and, at the same time, letting her know that someone understands how she feels.

As the story ended, a large group of doctors gathered around her door. Clearly and loudly Diane said, "Put that side up. Lock that door." The nurse said, "I'll see if they want anything. I don't think they are looking at you." The nurse then asked the physicians if they could move to another spot to talk and reassured Diane that they did not want to see her.

The doctor had dilated her esophagus that morning and the presence of the doctors was a reminder.
Asks for protection.

She then grabbed one book after the other for the nurse to read. "Read more stories," she said. When the nurse was leaving today, Diane said, "Leave that door open."

A real sign of acceptance. More trusting of her environment.

Day Three (eleventh hospital day)

A nurse's aide was trying to urge Diane to eat; Diane passively and quietly accepted the aide, although she refused to eat. When the nurse entered the room, Diane said, "Go away. Go away. Me wan' sleep. Go away." The doctor entered the room to take Diane to the treatment room for dilatation and she became terrified. She asked the nurse to put her in bed, put the side up, and lock the door. The nurse attempted to reassure her that the tube was going to help her throat get better, but understanding was impossible and anxiety extremely high.

Testing the interest of the nurse.

Asks for protection.

The nurse accompanied Diane to the treatment room and held her hand through the procedure. She fought through most of it and wilted when it was over. When the nurse picked her up to take her to her room, she weakly said, "Go room. Go bed. Wan's sleep."

A supporting presence in a time of stress.

Need to withdraw again and recooperate.

Once in her room, Diane crawled into bed and turned her face to the wall. She did not want to read or play. When she seemed to be sleeping, the nurse left the room.

Feels defeated.

When the nurse returned, Diane was sitting up in bed crying. The nurse said, "Diane is sad because she is in the hospital and the doctors must do painful things to her. She doesn't like it. But Diane is getting better and will go home soon. Pointing to the mineral oil on her stand, the nurse continued, "This medicine will also

Again trying to help her understand, even though the concepts are very abstract.

PROCESS RECORDINGS *(continued)*	COMMENTS *(continued)*
make Diane feel better." Diane reached over and drank it quickly. "Where's mommy. Mommy come back," she cried. Again the nurse reassured her that mommy loved her and would return that evening.	Help her understand the purpose of the medicine in simple terms. Needs constant reassurance that mommy will return.
After offering her the choice of several activities, including a ride in a cart, painting, reading, or the playroom, Diane suddenly said, "I wan' go to playroom."	Offer her the choices. First sign of wanting to leave the room.
She remained close by the nurse's side as she inspected the various activities of the playroom. She did not make any moves to play with the various toys and activities offered. Then a doctor came to look at her mouth. She moved closer to the nurse and cried. "He just wants to look at you. He won't hurt you. He wants to see how much better you are." Diane accepted the explanation and opened her mouth for inspection. When he left, she said, "I wan' paints." She painted very intently. After each picture, she asked about her mommy and was reassured that mommy loved her and would return soon.	Develops some trust. A good activity for release of emotions.
When she was finished painting, the nurse reminded her that it was time for the ointment that made her lips and finger get better. She followed the nurse through a group of doctors to the treatment room, where she applied the medicine herself with applicators.	More trusting. Independence allowed.

Day Four (twelfth hospital day)

Diane was sitting up in bed with her full liquid breakfast in front of her when the nurse arrived. Again when the nurse approached, Diane said, "Go away. Go away. Me sleepy. Go sleep." "I like you and I want to play with you. Maybe we could go to the playroom or paint or read." Diane responded, "I wan' go to playroom." The nurse agreed that they could do this as soon as Diane had finished her breakfast and had a bath.	Testing again. Setting limits.
When they arrived in the playroom, a doctor was casually sitting in a chair. Diane bravely followed the nurse into the room, eyeing the doctor suspiciously, but not verbalizing any fear. Accepting his presence, she again painted. She painted several paintings of various colors, stopping at times to inspect the messy paint on her fingers. "We'll wash that later," the nurse said. Soon she had paint on her face, arms, and gown. She was having a great time! Then the nurse told Diane that she was leav-	Trusting the environment more.

PROCESS RECORDINGS *(continued)*	COMMENTS *(continued)*
ing for a coffee break. Diane was quite content to stay alone with the other children. Upon the nurse's return, however, Diane watched her intently as she continued to paint.	Trust again is evident.
The nurse asked Diane if she wanted to take a picture to Jean; she readily agreed. Jean was crying when they entered the room and Diane looked worried. The nurse reminded Diane that Jean probably cried at home too when she was hungry. Diane nodded and smiled. Diane then gave her picture to her sister and ran into the hall where she grabbed a toy from the playpen to give to Jean. Then she intently inspected Jean's hand for lesions similar to her own. The nurse said, "Jean doesn't have sores on her fingers like you. Just on her mouth, and they are getting better. She will go home soon too." Diane then touched Jean's face and nose with her finger. They put Jean in bed and obtained another toy for Diane to give her. On the way back to the ward she said, "Me wan' to go back to the playroom."	Comparison to something at home makes it familiar. Is she inspecting Jean to learn more about her own injuries? Doesn't need to withdraw now.
When the nurse told Diane that it was time for her to leave that day, she was quite upset, and ran down the hall crying. The nurse reassured Diane that she would return the next day. Then Diane began to cry for her mommy. Again the nurse reassured her that mommy loved her very much and would come to visit at supper time.	Trust firmly established. The leaving of the nurse reminds her of an even more important loss. Supper is a more tangible time for her to remember, since the abstract concepts of time are not understandable at this age.

EVALUATION

An evaluation of the nursing approach based on the problem list and nursing care plan described earlier is an important part of nursing intervention. The nursing approach with Diane could be described as effective in that

1. Diane began to develop trust in her nurse, the doctors, and the environment, as shown by her ability to go to the playroom and walk past a group of doctors without trying to hide. Although not described in the process recordings, Diane also became more secure with her parents and was able to relate to them more effectively during their visits. She cried when they left, but trusted that they would return.
2. She began to assert her independence and autonomy by making requests and decisions for herself.

3. She was beginning to express herself through play activities or more directly by verbalization.
4. She seemed to have less need to withdraw into her room and crib.
5. She began to eat better and nutrition improved.
6. She slept and rested better.

It was not possible at this time to evaluate Diane's understanding of her illness and treatment measures, although attempts were made to help her understand broad concepts of the reasons for the hospitalization and treatments. Since the injury was largely internal (esophageal burn), she was not able to see it. A two-and-one-half-year-old has no concept about something inside his body which he cannot see—abstract thinking has not begun. Thus evaluation of her understanding of the injury and treatments was impossible at this time of the study.

STUDY GUIDE

Trust

1. How does a nurse develop trust with a patient?
2. How important is trust?

The Toddler

1. What are some of the sources of stress for a hospitalized toddler?
2. Why is it important for the nurse to help a toddler cope with separation?
3. What are some of the ways a nurse can help toddlers to cope with separation?
4. How can a nurse help the parents be more involved in helping their child cope with separation?
5. Why is independence important to the toddler?
6. How can a nurse encourage independence with toddlers?
7. When is dependence important?
8. How can a nurse assess the independence/dependence needs of toddlers?
9. Why is fear of bodily injury a big concern for a toddler?
10. How can a nurse help toddlers deal with this fear?
11. Why does a toddler need to understand his environment?
12. How can a nurse make the environment more familiar to a toddler?
13. What are some of the challenges in trying to communicate with a toddler?
14. How can a nurse communicate in nonverbal ways?
15. Who is a nurse's best resource when trying to communicate with a toddler?
16. How can play be used to help a child cope with illness and hospitalization?
17. Why is play important to the child?

18.   What are a nurse's concerns when giving care to a toddler and how does she deal with these concerns?

Accidents in Childhood

1.   What are the leading causes of death in children from birth to 14?
2.   How common are accidents?
3.   What are the developmental characteristics predisposing children to accidents for each age group (1 to 6 months; 7 to 12 months; 1 to 5 years; 6 to 12 years)?
4.   For each age group, what are some common accidents that occur?
5.   Suggest methods of prevention for each type of accident.
6.   What are the characteristics of accident-prone children?

Poisonings in Childhood

1.   How common are childhood poisonings?
2.   What symptoms are most frequently encountered in acute poisonings?
3.   What is the emergency treatment when poisoning is suspected?
4.   When is vomiting contraindicated?
5.   What is the function of poison control centers?
6.   How can poisonings be prevented?

SELECTED READINGS

J. M. Arena, "The Clinical Diagnosis of Poisoning," *The Pediatric Clinics of North America*, vol. 17, no. 3, August 1970, pp. 477–494.

C. Barnes, "Support of a Mother in the Care of a Child with Esophageal Lye Burns," *Nursing Clinics of North America*, vol. 4, no. 1, March 1969, pp. 53–57.

F. Blake, "A Search for Kathy's Problem," *International Journal of Nursing Studies*, vol. 2, pp. 125–136.

F. Blake, "In Quest of Hope and Autonomy," *Nursing Forum*, vol. 1, no. 1, Winter 1961–62, pp. 9–32.

C. T. Bombeck *et al.*, "Esophageal Trauma," *Surgical Clinics of North America*, vol. 52, no. 1, February 1972, pp. 219–230.

T. M. Cashman and H. C. Shirkey, "Emergency Management of Poisoning," *The Pediatric Clinics of North America*, vol. 17, no. 3, August 1970, pp. 525–534.

F. Erickson, "Nursing Care Based on Nursing Assessment," in Betty Bergerson (ed.), *Current Concepts in Clinical Nursing*, vol. 11, C. V. Mosby, St. Louis, 1969, pp. 171–177.

J. Hott, "Rx: Play P.R.N. in Pediatric Nursing," *Nursing Forum,* vol. IX, no. 3, 1970, pp. 288–309.

M. R. Miles, "Body Integrity Fears in a Toddler," *Nursing Clinics of North America,* vol. 4, no. 1, March 1969, pp. 39–51.

M. Petrillo, "Preventing Hospital Trauma in Pediatric Patients," *American Journal of Nursing,* vol. 68, July 1968, p. 1469.

M. Petrillo and S. Sanger, *Emotional Care of Hospitalized Children: An Environmental Approach,* "Play in the Hospital," pp. 99–133; "Guidelines for Working with Toddlers and Youngsters," pp. 141–143. J. B. Lippincott, Philadelphia, 1972.

R. G. Sherz, "Prevention to Childhood Poisoning: A Community Project," *Pediatric Clinics of North America,* vol. 17, no. 3, August 1970, pp. 713–727.

Marcia Thompson
eight and one-half years old

Cerebral Palsy/Chronic
Lorraine Wolf

The challenge of providing comprehensive nursing care is exemplified by working with children who have a disability at, or shortly after, birth. Resolution of the causative pathology during the episodic phase is of little value if physical crippling and mental or social maladaptation remain without continued intervention. Although the percentage of children with cerebral palsy is small, the following case study illustrates the numerous critical health care problems requiring long-term intervention.

CHIEF COMPLAINT

Marcia is an eight-and-one-half-year-old female referred to the Children's Rehabilitation Unit (CRU) following a visit to the Children and Youth (C&Y) Clinic. The mother states that Marcia has been very slow in development, and unable to walk, talk. or use her hands properly.

NURSING HISTORY

General Information

Marcia is the last of seven children and was born when her mother was thirty years old. She was delivered frank breech by double footling extraction. She failed to breathe spontaneously and was given artificial respiration for an undetermined period of time. It was apparently one hour before her normal breathing began. Her birth weight was 2.40 kg. She was observed in the hospital for seven days, resulting in a tentative diagnosis of cerebral damage.

Marcia was inactive in her early infancy. Her mother says, "She just laid on her back all day." She also failed to gain weight properly, and her weight at thirteen months was only 5.99 kg. At that time she was admitted to the hospital and the diagnostic impressions were spastic cerebral palsy, pneumonitis, and iron deficiency anemia.

Marcia continued to develop slowly, and at present is unable to walk, can speak only a few words, cannot feed or clothe herself, and has had no formal education. She is also far smaller than the normal child her age. Her mother says she is toilet trained, and she seems to play well with friends of all ages, although with no verbal communication on her part.

During years 4 to 7 Marcia's mother applied to special schools, hoping to enroll her in an educational situation, but there were no openings. Mrs. Thompson and her family moved to Kansas City about a year ago, and through her sister she became acquainted with the C&Y Clinic. Following the examination there a referral was made to the Children's Rehabilitation Unit.

Social Background

The mother was born in Kansas City, but when her parents separated, she moved to Indiana with her mother and siblings. She had her first child at age fifteen, and at age twenty had three children and was divorced from her first husband. She has four children by her second husband, Mr. Thompson. All of the children are normal except Marcia.

Mr. and Mrs. Thompson were separated many times, and finally Mr. Thompson did not return home. Mrs. Thompson has no idea where he is now, and he has never contributed to the support of his children. Mrs. Thompson receives assistance from the welfare department through the aid-to-dependent-children program.

NURSING ASSESSMENT

Developmental History

Language. Faulty articulation patterns are so severe that Marcia's speech is unintelligible. However, she has her own word for water—"owa"—and can nonverbally communicate her need to go to the bathroom. This articulation problem is due to poor muscle control; lack of mobility of tongue, lips, and jaw; and poor functioning of the palate.

Motor Coordination. There has been a history of Marcia's failure to thrive. For example, at 13 months she weighed 5.85 kg. Her physical growth at present is far below normal for her age, in both height and weight. Her head circumference is also more than two standard deviations below the mean.

According to the mother, Marcia did not sit unsupported until the age of six. She said her first words at the age of seven. She has never walked, although she can sit and crawl. At present she does not feed or dress herself. She has been toilet-trained since the age of two.

Social–Emotional Growth.   Mrs. Thompson states that Marcia enjoys watching TV and playing with dolls and children. Her six siblings help in her care. When I first met Marcia, she had a big smile, and communication was through those big brown eyes. Like any "normal" eight-year-old child, she is learning to find satisfaction with peers and other adults, but in different ways. She is just beginning to learn to play by herself, and she plays "beside" children rather than with them. Consultation with the mother reveals that Marcia frequently has temper tantrums at home—crying, kicking, and refusing to cooperate. Perhaps her temper tantrums are one way of showing others that she is an individual, whereas the nine-year-old, who has a similar need, is learning to participate in discussions and by communications. Unlike an eight-year-old, Marcia cannot take care of her own body needs. This may even double her frustrations.

Environmental History

The Thompsons live in a small duplex near the C&Y Clinic. The home is new and furnished with modern, plastic-coated furniture. The house is neat and clean, but dimly lit.

Mrs. Thompson states that Kansas City is her home. She said she moved back to Kansas City from Indiana after separating from her husband in hopes of finding some help for Marcia. She said that "people" in Indiana felt that Marcia could not be helped and that there was nothing anyone could do for her. Mrs. Thompson's sister (in Kansas City) suggested that Marcia be seen at the C&Y Clinic. This was done, resulting in a referral for the Children's Rehabilitation Unit evaluation.

Medical History

Physical Examination

General appearance. Marcia is an eight-and-one-half-year-old female, small for her age, appearing undernourished, spastic, nonambulatory, smiling, and cooperative. Height and weight are far below the third percentile for her age.

Head. Tympanic membranes are slightly dull with decreased reflexes but no acute inflammation was noted. Both upper canine teeth are missing and the right lower canine is also absent. Six-year molars are present. The eyes appear normal although the fundi were only briefly visualized.

Neck and chest. Within normal limit.

Cardiovascular. The P.M.I. is in the second intercostal space, higher than normally expected. No murmurs or thrills are noted.

Gastrointestinal. Masses are palpated. She has a stool once every 2 to 3 days. Stools are dark and firm with no evidence of blood.

Genitalia. Normal prepubertal female.

Urinary. Incontinent, on occasion urinates 3 to 4 times an hour during the day.

Musculoskeletal and neurologic. All four extremities are spastic and the adductors, hamstrings, and heel cords are especially tight. The metacarpalphalangeal joints are hyperextensible. There is atrophy of the muscles of the lower legs although the thigh muscles seem adequate. The child is able to sit alone with her knees sharply flexed and her lower legs lying along side her thighs. Deep tendon reflexes are absent in the knees and ankles, but appear to be normal in the upper extremities. Coordination is poor. Sensation appears intact. There is minimal drooling during the examination.

Diagnostic impression. Cerebral palsy (quadriplegia).

Other Assessments

Speech Evaluation.   Marcia, aged eight years, seven months, was seen for a speech and language evaluation as part of her total Children's Rehabilitation Unit workup. Mrs. Thompson reported that her daughter had speech problems and that her expressive vocabulary was limited to about five words. The mother thought that Marcia understood "pretty well." She reported that Marcia communicated by pointing, which she accompanied with vocalization. She stated that Marcia drooled constantly but had no difficulty swallowing, and that although she could chew hard food, she tended to swallow it without doing so.

Administration of the Peabody Picture Vocabulary Test, by Gail Butterfield in September 1969, indicated that Marcia's single-word comprehension was at a five year, one month level. Informal receptive testing at this evaluation indicated that she was functioning at about a four to five year level. She was able to execute commands of three commissions (tasks) but was unable to do four.

No formal articulation test was attempted. Marcia was able to imitate a few consonants in the initial position including /p/, /b/, /m/, /d/, /t/. She could imitate the vowels /a/ and /o/ but not /u/, /e/, /i/, /ai/. She could articulate consonant-vowel syllables using these consonants involved, but was unable to produce vowel-consonant syllables or vowel-consonant-vowel syllables. When imitating two-syllable combinations, she could not articulate them sequentially, but paused between syllables. Even these syllables were not clearly articulated, with a lax contact of the articulators. It appeared that she was unable to build up enough pressure for clear articulation of these sounds. Marcia was unable to imitate any fricative sounds.

Expressively, Marcia was able to imitate the names of a few simple objects such as ball, cup, spoon. However, her articulation was so poor that it was questionable if these words would be understood unless the context was known to the examiner. No spontaneous naming responses were intelligible.

Marcia's respiratory pattern was characterized by shallow inhalation and exhalation at about twenty-five per minute. This is slightly rapid. She was able to sustain phonation for about one second although she could phonate on command. She frequently phonated on both inspiration and expiration. She tended to extend her head backward to initiate voice, and the quality of tone was breathy and gravelly. Much mucous collected in her throat and she frequently coughed to clear it. This probably accounts for the gravelly voice characteristics. It appeared that her voice quality improved slightly and that phonation was easier to initiate with a flexed neck position.

Marcia was able to retract, purse, and close her lips on command. She could protrude her tongue to the vermillion of the lips but could not maintain that position. She was unable to either elevate or depress her tongue. At rest the tongue appeared to be in a retracted position, and involuntary movements were noted. At times the tongue was so far back in the oral cavity that Marcia almost choked. Velopharyngeal closure appeared to be adequate with good movement of the palate.

In summary, Marcie's speech is characterized by dysarthria. Her articulation is slow, requires effort, and is imprecise. Poor respiratory and laryngeal control interfere with production of good voice quality and efficient use of the breath stream. Poor tongue functioning contributes to the poor articulation skills; range, rate, and precision of movements are impaired. She is able to imitate a few consonant and vowel phonemes, but even these are imprecisely produced. This girl has had apparently no formal education or therapy, so it is difficult to estimate what skills she might have acquired with such training. Prognosis for further speech development is uncertain at this time. Speech therapy is recommended for a trial period to determine if Marcia's oral communication can be improved.

Hearing Evaluation.   *Note:* All decibel values are re: 22 dB CPS.

Marcia was given an audiological evaluation at this hospital. Because of the child's level of responsiveness, formal audiometric procedures were not possible. However, it was possible to gain useful information through more informal test procedures. The child was placed in a sound field and was stimulated with narrow bands of calibrated noise. Accurate localizing behavior was observed at 10 dB, in the sound field, for narrow band noises with center frequencies ranging from 250 Hz through 8000 Hz. Marcia was able to localize speech at 5-dB level in the sound field.

Because the child gave no intelligible verbal responses during the testing session, assessment of discrimination ability was not possible.

As a summary, results of the sound field test procedures indicate normal bilateral hearing sensitivity for both pure tones and speech.

Physical Therapy Evaluation. This eight-year-old girl was seen for evaluation of her gross motor function and development. She demonstrated obvious motor involvement. Upon examination, full ranges of motion were produced in the upper extremities. Bilateral contractures of the hip flexors, hamstrings, adductors, and heelcords were present. Athetoid movements of the upper extremities, neck, and face predominated. Drooling was most evident, as well as gutteral sounds with labored minimal vocabulary. She was happy and most cooperative throughout the evaluation.

Functionally, the child demonstrated some good skills. She was able to produce continuous rolling movement, get to a creep position, stand, and walk on her knees. She had exceptionally good balance in a knee-walk position, and it is reported by the mother that she "jumps" on her knees when she is angry and upset. She can assist in transfers, has relatively good understanding, and gives excellent cooperation.

Her hand activity is only fair because of the distorting athetoid movements, although she does have fair aim in reaching and some grasp-release accuracy. Solid objects are handled much better than food, which she readily crushes.

The functional level demonstrated by this child, who has apparently had no formal therapy or academic programming, is strikingly good. In my estimation she is an excellent candidate for a Children's Rehabilitation Unit placement, in association with the allied services provided through psychology, physical therapy, occupational therapy, and speech.

NURSING INTERVENTION

PROBLEM		NURSING INTERVENTION (*directing or teaching parents*)
Communication		
1. Need for understandable speech	1.0	Provide correct words for objects and increase vocabulary as tolerated
	1.1	Encourage verbal play but do not frustrate
	1.2	Accept child's approximate motion, but offer correct pattern each time
	1.3	Use peanut butter on roof of child's mouth to increase facility of tongue
	1.4	Refer for speech therapy if possible
2. Need for expanding non-verbal communication	2.0	Watch eyes and body tension or motion for understanding, and reward with praise

GOAL: To aid in Marcia's socialization and independence and in maximizing educational experience.

PROBLEM (cont'd)	NURSING INTERVENTION (directing or teaching parents—cont'd)

Neuromuscular—Learning muscular skills

1. Inability to do balanced sitting

   1.0 Undertake passive exercises of extremities
   1.1 Train child on straddle toys. Guide legs in slow bicycle movements
   1.2 Assist in rolling on a large ball to develop ability to catch herself and to fall properly

2. Not walking

   2.0 Undertake passive range of motion exercises of lower extremities
   2.1 Support in standing position for short periods of time, several times daily

3. Spastic grasp

   3.0 Offer materials of different texture to stimulate tactile and kinesthetic input
   3.1 Exercise elbow extensors to increase reach and grasp
   3.2 Exercise of forearm supinators and wrist extensors for functional grasp motions
   3.3 Release thumb from palm and replace it with a toy several times a day

GOAL: To maximize Marcia's physical potential; to move toward independence.

Self-help skills

1. Inability to bathe self

   1.0 Give child washcloth and guide hand in washing movements
   1.1 Reward efforts to maintain good hygiene

2. Inability to feed self

   2.0 Offer small amounts (one or two swallows) from covered cup. When offering cup, place both child's hands on cup and guide
   2.1 Offer finger foods, allowing time for adequate mastication
   2.2 Fit with spoon and wrist stabilizer and allow child to try self-feeding with soft foods
   2.3 Include child in table talk

3. Not dressing self

   3.0 Dress slowly to avoid pain. Name body parts and clothing while dressing
   3.1 Use clothes that fasten in front, elastic bands in slacks and skirts, which are easier for child
   3.2 Use training board to teach child to button, zip, and tie

4. Poor dental hygiene

   4.0 Provide child with own toothbrush
   4.1 Guide hand in brushing teeth

PROBLEM (cont'd)	NURSING INTERVENTION (directing or teaching parents—cont'd)
5. Occasional "accidents" in bowel and bladder control	5.0 Watch for nonverbal signs (grimace or sounds) 5.1 Assist to bathroom and allow child to do as much as possible for self. Praise efforts 5.2 Protect at night if unable to call or get up alone

GOAL: To develop independence in the activities of daily living to the degree Marcia is capable and to aid in her vocalization process.

Social development

1. Primarily parallel and isolated play	1.0 Support hands and arms and guide in interactive games, i.e., "peek-a-boo," "button-button," and checkers 1.1 Offer light-weight magazines that can be torn into confetti collages by two or more children 1.2 Include in activities such as finger painting
2. Temper tantrums	2.0 Introduce tolerance for tension and discomfort in meeting needs slowly 2.1 Show approval and give praise for desirable behavior; correct errors in behavior immediately 2.2 Ignore temper tantrums except to provide physical protection 2.3 Set up alternatives for child to choose from (clothes, food, games) 2.4 Avoid bribing or teasing; be consistent in expectations, rewards, and punishments

GOAL: To foster appropriate interpersonal social contacts from which Marcia may draw for her own maturation and satisfaction.

Family (one-parent family)

1. Emotional needs for Marcia and siblings not adequately being met	1.0 Counsel mother to reevaluate and reset goals for Marcia to bring expectations in line with Marcia's potential 1.1 Reinforce mother's parenting ability 1.2 Involve siblings with Marcia's care, i.e., developing creative ways to help Marcia accomplish self-care 1.3 Refer other siblings for counseling if behavior problems continue 1.4 Assist in adapting child-rearing practices to Marcia

PROBLEM *(cont'd)*	NURSING INTERVENTION *(directing or teaching parents—cont'd)*	
	1.5	Support consultation with siblings in understanding Marcia's potential and limitations
2. Costly, long-term medical, surgical, and educational intervention needed for Marcia	2.0	Refer to Crippled Children's Commission for financial assistance in medical and surgical care
	2.1	Support mother in seeking placement in special education for Marcia
3. Mother unable to work	3.0	Refer to welfare caseworker and support for on-the-job training

GOAL: To maintain family continuity and move toward social and financial independence.

STUDY GUIDE

1. Various authors state that the etiology is unknown in 25 to 30 percent of the cases of cerebral palsy.
   a. Discuss the seven major etiological factors occurring during the preparanatal period that have been identified for 90 percent of the known cases.
   b. Based on the above discussion, define the nurse's role in prevention and early detection of cerebral palsy.
2. Marcia was diagnosed as having cerebral damage shortly after birth. In many children, however, it is not detected until they are one to two years old.
   a. Review the neurological responses (reflexes) normally present at birth. Identify those that would be critical in determining cerebral irritation or damage. At what age would the presence or absence of these reflexes be ominous?
   b. Review the developmental milestones of the first two years of life. Why is it important to assess and record this data on all children? On high-risk children?
3. Although Marcia has never had a convulsion, this is a common sequela of cerebral insult.
   a. List the drugs most often used for the control of seizures with infants and children. Dosages, side effects, and long-term therapy problems should be discussed in terms of both hospital and home care.
   b. What safety precautions need to be employed in the hospital and at home to protect the child subject to seizures?
4. Children such as Marcia may appear to be mentally retarded because of

their inability to communicate, awkward movements, facial grimaces, and drooling. Developmental assessments on standard tests, such as the Denver Developmental Screening Test, are not possible in the traditional manner.

    a. Discuss two or three different definitions for mental retardation, specifically looking at developmental milestones.

    b. In reviewing the physical manifestations of cerebral palsy, what normal processes of learning may have been omitted or underdeveloped?

5. Behavioral and emotional development are critical to determining the child's adaptation and ability to function in school and society.

    a. What verbal and nonverbal clues should the nurse look for in the parents' and/or siblings' interactions that indicate potential unresolved problems?

    b. What behaviors exhibited by the child indicate inappropriate responses in emotional development?

6. Subsequent to the case presentation Marcia had a bilateral adductor tenotomy and hamstring release.

    a. What other surgical procedures are commonly employed to enhance motor development? At what ages are they most successful?

    b. What special preparation and intervention should be incorporated in the hospital care for these patients? What concerns are most often expressed by the family?

7. Education and training are essential to assist children with cerebral palsy in finding a useful and rewarding place in society.

    a. Define the nurse's role in anticipatory guidance of parents and child for this experience.

    b. What resources are available in the community and state? Are preschool programs and special education classes available? What is the nurse's role in these programs?

8. As Marcia moves toward adolescence, she will develop normal heterosexual interests.

    a. Discuss the "myths" about the sexual development and activity of physically handicapped and/or mentally retarded adolescents.

    b. What intervention will be necessary to help Marcia deal with her body image, severe limitations in communication skills, and learning activities of daily living in order to prevent frustration and social isolation?

    c. When should this intervention be implemented?

SELECTED READINGS

B. Andrews *et al.*, "Cerebral Palsy: My Baby Is Slow," *Patient Care*, vol. 6, March 30, 1970.

K. Barnard and M. Powell, *Teaching the Mentally Retarded Child: A Family Care Approach*, C. V. Mosby, St. Louis, 1972.

E. Blumenthal *et al.*, "Guiding the Family of the Handicapped Child," *Patient Care*, vol. 6, March 30, 1972.

W. Cruickshank, *Cerebral Palsy: Its Individual and Community Problem*, Syracuse University Press, Syracuse, N.Y., 1966.

M. Debuskey, *The Chronically Ill Child and His Family*, Charles C Thomas, Springfield, Ill., 1970, chaps. 1 and 2.

E. Denhoff, *Cerebral Palsy—The Preschool Years*, Charles C Thomas, Springfield, Ill., 1967.

Nancy Finnie, *Handling the Young Cerebral Palsied Child at Home*, E. P. Dutton, New York, 1970.

Karl C. Garrison and Dewey G. Force, *The Psychology of Exceptional Children*, Ronald Press, New York, 1959, pp. 360–384.

Una Haynes, *A Development Approach to Case Finding with Special Reference to Cerebral Palsy, Mental Retardation, and Related Disorders*, Department of Health, Education, and Welfare, Children's Bureau, Washington, D.C., 1970.

K. S. Holt, *Assessment of Cerebral Palsy*, Lloyd Luke, London, 1965, chap. 1.

Wendell Johnson *et al.*, *Speech Handicapped School Children*, Harper & Row, Chicago, 1967.

Sidney Keats, *Operative Orthopedics in Cerebral Palsy*, Charles C Thomas, Springfield, Ill., 1970.

Dorothy Marlow, *Textbook of Pediatric Nursing*, W. B. Saunders, Philadelphia, 1965, pp. 398–403.

P. Pother, "Therapeutic Handling of the Severely Handicapped Child," *Nursing Clinics of North America*, vol. 5, September 1970.

M. A. Smolock, "The Nurse's Role in Rehabilitation of the Handicapped Child," *Nursing Clinics of North America*, vol. 5, September 1970.

K. F. Swaiman and F. S. Wright, *Neuro-Muscular Diseases of Infancy and Childhood*, Charles C Thomas, Springfield, Ill., 1970, chap. 1.

James Wolf, *The Results of Treatment in Cerebral Palsy*, Charles C Thomas, Springfield, Ill., 1969.

Todd Martin

nine years old

Cystic Fibrosis/ Acute and Chronic

Jeanne R. Schott

Todd is a small, very thin, nine-year-old boy with a protuberant abdomen and spindly extremities who has been diagnosed with cystic fibrosis since he was two and one-half years old. He appears short for his age and has always been well behind other children his own age in height and weight—near the tenth percentile in weight and below the third percentile in height on the growth chart.

Todd and his family live on a farm eight miles from a small town in western Kansas. Mr. Martin is a farmer and in off-season works part time for a farm machinery company. Mrs. Martin, a housewife, is kept very busy caring for Todd and his two normal brothers, six and eleven years old. Since he was two and one-half years old, Todd has been going to the cystic fibrosis clinic for regular checkups.

A great deal of equipment and medicine is necessary to carry out Todd's treatment in the home. He sleeps in a small, waterproof room (the walls are painted with rubber paint), which his parents built on to the house. The humidifier is left on all night, and he receives IPPB treatments twice a day. These are administered by his mother. In addition, he is receiving enzymes and antibiotics orally in large, daily doses. This medicine and equipment is paid for by the Cystic Fibrosis Fund of the Kansas Board of Health. The hospital bills from Todd's four hospital admissions are covered by Blue Cross–Blue Shield.

Todd's parents have made an ideal adjustment to their son's illness and are quite willing and anxious to learn of any new treatments necessary for his care.

PAST MEDICAL HISTORY

Prenatal, Natal, and Neonatal

Gestation and birth were uncomplicated. There was full-term, spontaneous delivery, and birth weight was 3.30 kg. The child was reported to be cyanotic at birth.

Age One Year

The child had a large appetite but would vomit; his weight was 8.10 kg (3.15 kg behind his other two siblings at the same age); he had foamy, foul-smelling stools, increased sweating, and severe chest colds.

Age Eighteen Months

Todd began talking and walking.

Age Two and One-Half Years

Cystic fibrosis was diagnosed by a local medical doctor by means of the sweat test and the analysis of enzymes from duodenal secretions (Todd lacked trypsin and amylase). Treatment included

1. Cotazyme, one/meal
2. Vitamin A, 50,000 units/day
3. Declomycin, 4 tsp./day
4. Regular diet with skim milk.

Age Four

Todd had herniorraphy and appendectomy.

Age Five

Sweat electrolytes were repeated and were positive for cystic fibrosis. Chest x rays showed no evidence of fibrosis in the lungs. Physical developmental lag was more apparent.

Age Eight

Todd was hospitalized with pneumonia for one week in August and treated with penicillin. He was rehospitalized for pneumonia in September for one week in a local hospital.

In October Todd's condition was worse and he was referred to the Cystic Fibrosis Clinic. Signs and symptoms included

1.   Early morning coughing spells
2.   Coughing all day—sputum light yellow
3.   Foamy, mustard-colored stools
4.   Stomach pains, particularly after hot, spicy foods.

Todd was sent home on the following treatment plan:

1.   Inhalation therapy with Neosynephrine and Mucomyst
2.   Postural drainage
3.   Mist tent at night
4.   Cotazyme with meals and snacks
5.   Water-soluble multivitamins
6.   Normal diet with emphasis on increased protein and low fat
7.   Antibiotics for signs of infection
8.   Expectorant p.r.n.

Age Nine

Todd was admitted to the hospital for treatment of pneumonia in September. Signs and symptoms included

1.   tired most of summer
2.   foul-smelling, loose, mushy stools
3.   anorexia
4.   coughing
5.   pallor
6.   weakness
7.   low-grade fever (100°F).

PHYSICAL EXAM ON ADMISSION

Weight: 20 kg, height 48½ in. Malnourished, small, thin boy in no acute distress

HEENT: emaciated facies—otherwise within normal limits

Chest, lungs: crepitant rale in left anterior chest; chest hyperresonant to percussion diffusely

Abdomen: protuberant, no organomegaly

Back and extremities: minimal cyanosis and clubbing noted bilaterally

Genitalia: herniorraphy scar on right side; skin otherwise clear

Neurological: grossly intact

Urinalysis: within normal limits

Histo and TB skin tests: negative

Nose and throat culture: pseudomonas and staph coagulase positive

Chest x ray: bronchopneumonia including the left-lower and left-middle lung area and involving the right midchest and atelectasis of the right upper lobe.

BLOOD TESTS

C.B.C.	Hg	Hct.	W.B.C.		
Initial	12.6	38	20,670	*Segs* 81 / *Mono* 4	*Lymphs* 50 / *Retic* 2.8
Last	11.2	36	8,760	*Segs* 74 / *Monos* 7	*Lymphs* 17 / *Eos* 2
					Platelets Adequate

HOSPITAL PROGRESS (9/11–9/28)

Treatment consisted of

1. Prostaphlin, 250 mg I.V. q. 8 h.
2. Polymyxin B, 52 mg I.V. q. 12 h.
3. IPPB with 3 cc Mucomyst mixed with ½ cc 1% Neosynephrine
4. postural drainage q.i.d.
5. multivitamins, 1 tablet t.i.d.
6. Cotazyme, 4 tablets before each meal and 2 tablets before each snack
7. I.V. fluids: 400 cc D_5W
   q. 12 h.   100 cc RL
              10 meq KCl
8. low-fat diet.

Todd was essentially afebrile throughout the hospital course. He was put on Prostaphlin and Polymyxin B intravenously and was kept on this for about two weeks. This treatment was based on the positive cultures for pseudomonas and coagulase positive staph. Todd clinically responded very well and his chest was much clearer at time of dismissal. However, it was felt at this time that lung congestion and pneumonia would probably be a chronic problem.

Todd was discharged with the following orders

1. oxytetracycline, 250 mg q.i.d.
2. IPPB with Neosynephrine and Mucomyst—family able to get Bennett through a child health center
3. 40-G fat diet—mother instructed
4. continue mist tent at night with 3% N.S. in propylene glycol
5. bronchial drainage q.i.d.
6. Cotazyme (2–5) with meals and snacks (2)
7. vitamins E (50 mg) and K (3 mg) plus multivitamins t.i.d.
8. return to cystic fibrosis clinic in two weeks.

Todd will be followed by the local physician and the physician at the cystic fibrosis clinic.

STUDY GUIDE

Goal One

To clear the tracheobronchial tree of retained mucopurulent secretion.
Questions to consider:
1. Why is this goal important in relation to the pathophysiology of this disease?
2. What methods can be used to thin and moisten viscid secretions? Why are they used? What are the nursing responsibilities?
3. What observations indicate a need for measures to clear the tracheo-bronchial tree?
4. What methods should be used to clear these secretions from the tracheo-bronchial tree? What are the nursing responsibilities?
5. What observations indicate success in clearing the tracheobronchial tree of secretions?
6. Todd's problem: Todd would not expectorate mucous; he preferred to swallow it. Why might Todd prefer to swallow mucous? How could we help Todd to accept the need to expectorate instead of swallow?

Goal Two

To prevent infection, particularly respiratory infection.
Questions to consider:
1. Why is Todd prone to infection?
2. What symptoms and problems did Todd have prior to his last hospitalization that were indications of infection?

3. What kind of guidance do Todd and his family need in relation to this goal?
4. What kind of planning does one need to consider in the hospital setting to prevent infection?

Goal Three

To help the child maintain adequate nutrition.
Questions to consider:
1. What are the normal nutritional needs of a school-age boy?
2. What are the particular needs of Todd in relation to his illness?
3. What symptoms should be observed in relation to Todd's nutritional status?
4. What kind of guidance should be given to this family regarding Todd's nutritional needs?
5. Todd's problem: He was a very poor eater, consuming mostly carbohydrates. What should be the plan of care during hospitalization to help Todd eat better?

Goal Four

To prevent fatigue by promoting good patterns of rest and sleep.
Questions to consider:
1. After reading Todd's history, why do you think fatigue may have been a problem during his last hospitalization?
2. What might be the nursing intervention for Todd to promote good patterns of rest and sleep?

Goal Five

To promote physical comfort and good hygiene.
Questions to consider:
1. Why would skin care be of prime importance in promoting comfort for Todd?
2. Todd's teeth were very tartared, brown, and unsightly. Why might his teeth be like this? What are the implications for nursing care?

Goal Six

To help the child cope with the illness and the medical treatment.
Questions to consider:
1. What are the particular stresses for a school-age child, like Todd, with a long-term illness?
2. What are the implications for nursing intervention?

Goal Seven

To help the child achieve his developmental tasks.
Questions to consider:
1. What are Todd's developmental needs?
2. What kind of planning should be done in the hospital and at home to help Todd master this stage of development?
3. Todd's problem: He was concerned about missing so many days from school (30 to 40). He had received A's and B's prior to the illness and and was worried about future grades. How might the nurse deal with Todd's concerns about school and his future grades?

Goal Eight

To help parents and family to face the diagnosis and to carry out the prescribed regimen in an optimistic manner.
Questions to consider:
1. What might be the role of nurses in the hospital setting and the home setting to assist this family?
2. What are the financial burdens for this type of family?
3. Why might parents feel guilty?
4. What affect might a chronic illness like cystic fibrosis have on the siblings of a family? What are the implications for nursing intervention?
5. What resources are available to help a family such as Todd's?

SELECTED READINGS

M. A. Crate, "Nursing Functions in Adaptation to Chronic Illness," *American Journal of Nursing*, vol. 65, no. 10, October 1965, pp. 72–76.

F. Erikson, "When 6–12 Year Olds Are Ill," *Nursing Outlook*, vol. 13, no. 7, July 1965, pp. 48–50.

N. Forbes, "The Nurse and Genetic Counseling," *Nursing Clinics of North America*, vol. 1, no. 4, December 1966, pp. 137–142.

F. C. Fraser, "Genetic Counseling," *Hospital Practice*, vol. 6, no. 1, January 1971, pp. 49–56.

C. Gips, "The Interpretation and Misinterpretation by Hospitalized School Age Children of Being Sick: Implications for Nursing," *ANA Nurses Convention*, vol. 11, no. 15, 1962, pp. 13–20.

A. Hargreaves, "Emotional Problems of Patients with Respiratory Disease," *Nursing Clinics of North America*, vol. 3, no. 3, September 1968, pp. 481–482.

M. Kurihara, "Postural Drainage, Clapping, and Vibrating," *American Journal of Nursing*, vol. 65, no. 11, November 1965, pp. 76–79.

V. Lockhart *et al.*, "An Interdisciplinary Approach to Cystic Fibrosis," *Inhalation Therapy*, vol. 15, no. 2, April 1970, pp. 34–40.

D. R. Marlowe, *Textbook of Pediatric Nursing*, W. B. Saunders, Philadelphia, 1969, pp. 328–333, and pp. 563–566.

R. S. Mendelsohn, "Broadening the Horizons of Pediatric Practice: Problems of Management of Chronic Diseases as Exemplified by Cystic Fibrosis," *Clinical Pediatrics*, vol. 9, no. 11, November 1970, pp. 638–641.

H. S. Mitchell *et al.*, *Cooper's Nutrition in Health and Disease*, J. B. Lippincott, Philadelphia, 1968, pp. 380–381.

B. J. Rosenstein, "Cystic Fibrosis of the Pancreas: Impact on Family Functioning," in Matthew Debuskey (ed.), *The Chronically Ill Child and His Family*, Charles C. Thomas, Springfield, Ill., 1970, pp. 23–32.

H. Schwachman and Kon-Tail Khan, "Cystic Fibrosis," in Harry C. Shirkey (ed.), *Pediatric Therapy*, C. V. Mosby, St. Louis, 1968, pp. 576–596.

S. Stadnyk and N. Bindschadler, "A Camp for Children with Cystic Fibrosis," *American Journal of Nursing*, vol. 70, no. 8, August 1970, pp. 1691–1693.

V. B. Tisza, "Management of the Parents of the Chronically Ill Child," *American Journal of Orthopsychiatry*, vol. 32, no. 53, January 1962.

A. Tropauer *et al.*, "Psychological Aspects of the Care of Children with Cystic Fibrosis," *American Journal of Diseases of Children*, vol. 119, no. 5, May 1970, pp. 424–432.

Review Normal Growth and Development of the School Age Child.

Mark Davis
nine years old

Acute Lymphocytic Leukemia/ Acute and Chronic
Jeanne R. Schott

Mark was a nine-year-old boy when he was initially diagnosed with leukemia in August of 1969. Three to four weeks prior to admission to the hospital for diagnosis, Mark had a cold, developed right knee joint pains, and limped for two days. Two weeks prior to that, Mark had right shoulder pain, difficulty extending his right arm, and right ankle pain. He was taken to a private doctor, who prescribed aspirin four times daily for five days. No other medications were given. Mark continued to be lethargic with no relief of symptoms and was admitted to a private hospital. The physical exam showed cervical lymphadenopathy and a palpable spleen. The complete blood count at this time showed a hemoglobin of 9.9 percent, hematocrit of 30 percent, white blood cells of 1,500 with 82 percent lymphocytes, 16 percent segmenters, and 2 percent monocytes. The bone marrow showed a predominance of immature lymphocytes, and Mark was diagnosed with acute lymphocytic leukemia. Protocol induction therapy with prednisone and vincristine was recommended and Mark was transferred to this hospital to begin treatment.

Mark was a full-term, spontaneous delivery. He was healthy at birth, with a birth weight of 3.90 kg. His psychomotor development has been normal. Mark had had chickenpox and measles when he was three years old and has had no other childhood diseases except for an occasional cold. His tonsils are intact and he has had no surgical procedures done.

Mark's parents, Mr. Davis, thirty-seven, and Mrs. Davis, thirty-four, are living and well. His two siblings, both boys, eleven and thirteen, are also living and well. There is no history of diabetes in the family except for one maternal grandmother, who had the adult onset type. There is no history of leukemia or blood dyscrasias in the family. Mr. Davis is employed by an airline company and will pay for the hospitalization by insurance and by his own funds.

The physical exam at this hospital revealed that the head, eyes, ears, nose, and throat were unremarkable except for extreme pale mucosa and conjunctiva. The neck was supple with no lymphadenopathy and thyromegaly. The chest and lungs were clear. The heart had a normal sinus rhythm with no murmurs and no cardiomegaly. The abdomen was flat with no hepatomegaly. The spleen was three fingerbreadths below the left costal margin. The extremities were unremarkable. The nervous system was intact.

Mark's urinalysis was normal. His complete blood count showed a hemoglobin of 9.1 percent, hematocrit of 26 percent, and a decreased white blood cell count. The chest and right shoulder x rays were negative. A bone marrow examination done at this hospital showed acute lymphocytic leukemia.

Induction therapy was begun September 26 with 2 mg of vincristine intravenously weekly and 60 mg of prednisone daily. Mark tolerated the medications well and was hospitalized until the blast forms in the peripheral smear decreased. He was discharged on October 3 to be followed up in the clinic. His repeat complete blood count at that time showed a 9.9 percent hemoglobin, 28.5 percent hematocrit, 5,200 white blood count, and adequate platelets. There were 3.8 percent reticulocytes.

CLINIC VISITS

10/14
Mark is active and cheerful. No petechiae, bleeding, or bruising noted. No lymphadenopathy or splenomegaly. Pale and afebrile. Mark is complaining of a sore throat today. Mild hyperemia of the throat seen with no exudate. Third dose of vincristine given intravenously. Continue prednisone 60 mg daily.

10/21
Mark is asymptomatic and gaining weight. No lymphadenopathy, hepatosplenomegaly, or skin lesions. Fourth dose of vincristine given intravenously. Prednisone continued. Hemoglobin 11.8 g percent, hematocrit 36 percent, white blood count 8,570, segmenters 84 percent, lymphocytes 15 percent, platelets 402,000.

10/28
Mark remains asymptomatic with no loss of hair or hepatosplenomegaly. Fifth dose of vincristine given intravenously. Prednisone continued. Hemoglobin 11.9 g percent, hematocrit 36 percent, white blood count 7,860, segmenters 70 percent, lymphocytes 17 percent, platelets 345,000.

11/3
Bone marrow aspiration done. Normal results.

11/11
Methotrexate, 20 mg orally biweekly (Tuesday and Saturday) begun.

11/25

Mark is active and alert with cushinoid facies. He is afebrile with no pallor, lymphadenopathy, hepatomegaly, or bruises. He did have some pain in his left knee about a week ago but there is no pain now. Mark has been complaining of painless sores in his mouth for the last three to four days. On examination, multiple small, shallow white ulcers were seen in both inner sides of his cheeks. The prednisone has been tapered off. It was felt at this time that Mark's leukemia was in remission and that his mouth ulcers were secondary to methotrexate toxicity. Mark will continue on methotrexate 20 mg biweekly. Hemoglobin 12.9 g percent, hematocrit 39 percent, white blood count 9,070, segmenters 82 percent, lymphocytes 14 percent, platelets 226,000.

12/30

Mark's appetite has decreased and he is complaining of early morning nausea. He also has an occasional brief mild headache. He skipped four doses of methotrexate two to three weeks ago because of oral ulcerations. At the present time he has no ulcers in his mouth. The leukemia remains in remission. Continue methotrexate 20 mg biweekly. Hemoglobin 12.8 g percent, hematocrit 38 percent, white blood count 5,000, segmenters 43 percent, lymphocytes 42 percent, platelets 271,000.

2/10/70

Mark has done well since his last clinic visit. He complained of a headache twice in January. These were short in duration and relieved by aspirin. Last night he complained of a sore in his mouth. He had not had oral ulceration since December. The physical exam showed a somewhat pale boy with no lymphadenopathy or hepatomegaly. He did have moderate tenderness on palpation over the spleen. The spleen was not palpable. There was a small ulcer with a white base and erythematous ridge on the lower lip. Leukemia is in remission. Plan to hold the methotrexate dose today to see the effect on the oral membrane ulcer, then return to methotrexate biweekly.

3/24

Mark is doing very well with no complaints. Continue methotrexate biweekly. Hemoglobin 12.5 g percent, white blood count 2,960, platelets 176,000.

5/12

Doing very well except for some nausea and vomiting. Leukemia in remission. Continue methotrexate. Hemoglobin 12.7 g percent, hematocrit 37 percent, white blood count 3,680, segmenters 24 percent, lymphocytes 72 percent, platelets 105,000.

6/12
Mark has been complaining of swelling in the left groin for the past two days and has been limping. He is afebrile and does not appear toxic. The physical exam revealed a tender, enlarged, mobile lymph node in the left groin. He has multiple skin lesions (some infected) on the cheek, trunk, and extremities. It was felt that the skin lesions were impetigo and that Mark also had infective lymphadenitis. He was placed on Dynapen every six hours for ten days and was to begin pHisoHex soaks. The next two doses of methotrexate were to be omitted and Mrs. Davis was to call the clinic in two to three days.

6/16
Mark was seen in the emergency room with chest and back pain. Two days ago Mark had upper thoracic back pain which responded to aspirin. Today he began complaining of substernal pain. His oral temperature was 38.2°C. The impetigo was clearing. He had no splenomegaly or hepatomegaly. There was tenderness to palpation of T_5 and T_6. He was sent home.

SECOND HOSPITAL ADMISSION

6/20
Mark was admitted to the hospital with fever and joint pain. He was doing well until ten days ago, when his father noted that he was lethargic and had bruises scattered over both extremities. The next day he had a tender lump in the left groin. Mark has continued to have malaise and a decreased appetite. Although the impetigo has cleared up, he has recurrent discomfort in both knees, both hips, and the mid-back region radiating around the chest.

On physical exam, Mark presented as a pale, alert child in no acute distress. The optic discs were not sharp but there is no diopter change between the disc and the remaining fundus. The visual fields were normal. Mark has had headaches during school lasting about an hour; these have caused the top of his head to become numb. The left tympanic membrane is red with a decreased light reflex. The right tympanic membrane is normal. Mark's throat is inflamed, his gums are pale, and there may be gum hypertrophy in the right cheek area of denuded mucosa. The abdomen is soft with no masses. The liver is palpable one centimeter below the right costal margin. On inspiration, the spleen is down 3 to 4 cm below the left costal margin. The axillary nodes are prominent and tender and the inguinal nodes are large and painful. Pain is evoked with any leg movement. Mark has had no constipation, melena, hematemesis, diarrhea, or frank blood in his stool. He has had no sudden weight loss and did have a marked gain in weight after prednisone was instituted. He also had increased irritability after prednisone was withdrawn.

On this admission the parents verbalized they were having trouble with Mark's two brothers resenting all the attention that Mark was getting. Mr. and Mrs. Davis have not discussed Mark's disease with Mark or his two brothers. Mr. and Mrs. Davis also said that Mark does not get along in school with his peers, as his teacher treats him specially. Mark is not doing as well in school as he had in the past. He seems to have an indifferent attitude toward school and does not want to go to school. At this time Mr. and Mrs. Davis were encouraged to join a parent group composed of parents of children with terminal illnesses which was under the guidance of a child psychiatrist.

The urinalysis, glucose, blood, urea, nitrogen, and creatinine were normal. A spinal tap was done and 8 cc of spinal fluid was removed. Opening pressure was 266 cm of water and closing pressure was 160 cm of water. The cerebral spinal fluid revealed 145 white blood cells, 55 red blood cells with 2 neutrophils and 98 mononuclears. The spinal fluid glucose was 49 mg percent and the protein was 26 mg percent. These results were quite suggestive of central nervous system infiltration of leukemia and Mark's sudden relief, although short, may be due to release of cerebral spinal fluid pressure. Blood and urine cultures showed no growth. There was normal flora in the throat culture. The complete blood count on admission revealed a hemoglobin of 12 g percent, 4,290 white blood count with 14 percent segmenters, and 74 percent lymphocytes. The bone marrow aspiration was interpreted as acute lymphocytic leukemia. X rays were taken of the areas of bone discomfort. They showed typical patterns of leukemia in the bones of the knee joints, particularly the tibia and femur.

Mark spiked several temperatures while hospitalized and blood cultures were drawn. These were negative for pathogens. The bone marrow aspiration showed the presence of an exacerbation of acute lymphocytic leukemia, and induction therapy was begun three days after admission (June 23). The drugs used were vincristine, 2 mg intravenously weekly and 60 mg of prednisone daily. Mark was discharged June 24 to be followed in the clinic.

CLINIC VISITS

6/30

Mark continues to be lethargic and had one headache yesterday. He has had double vision each night since he returned from the hospital. Two days after dismissal Mark developed a cold, cough, and sore throat. He has a few new bruises and is afebrile. He has had no vomiting, constipation, or alopecia. His appetite is increased but is not excessive. The second dose of vincristine was given intravenously. Prednisone was continued 60 mg daily. Hemoglobin 12.4 g percent, hematocrit 35 percent, white blood count 2,700, segmenters 49 percent, lymphocytes 47 percent, platelets 125,000, reticulocytes 0.2 percent.

7/7

Mark has been complaining of body aches for the past two days. There was no lymphadenopathy, the liver was felt on deep inspiration, the spleen was not palpable. The third dose of vincristine was given intravenously. Prednisone was continued. Hemoglobin 11.2 g percent, hematocrit 32.6 percent, white blood count 5,100, segmenters 56 percent, lymphocytes 30 percent, platelets 205,000.

7/14

Mark is complaining of an occasional body ache and has some loss of hair. There were no other findings. The fourth dose of vincristine was given intravenously. Prednisone was continued. Hemoglobin 10.3 g percent, hematocrit 30.5 percent, white blood count 4,400, segmenters 52 percent, lymphocytes 46 percent, platelets 183,000.

7/21

Mark has gained two pounds since his last clinic visit. Otherwise the exam is essentially unchanged. The fifth dose of vincristine was given intravenously. Prednisone was continued. Hemoglobin 10.2 g percent, hematocrit 26.3 percent, white blood count 6,600, segmenters 63 percent, lymphocytes 33 percent, platelets 196,000.

7/28

Mark is doing well. He has gained three pounds since his last visit. There has been no bleeding or central nervous system symptoms. The sixth dose of vincristine was given intravenously today. Prednisone was continued.

8/3

Bone marrow was performed and shows remission of acute lymphocytic leukemia. Mark was begun on 75 mg of 6 mercaptopurine (6 MP) daily.

8/25

Acute lymphocytic leukemia is in remission. Mark is asymptomatic at present. Continue 6 mercaptopurine.

9/8

Mark has been on 6 mercaptopurine daily for five weeks. He has had chest pain for four days, which is worse with deep breathing. He has a slight cough but denies having a sore throat. Last night Mark had a fever of 38.6°C, but it was normal this morning. Hemoglobin 10.6 g percent, white blood count 2,370, platelets 203,000.

THIRD HOSPITAL ADMISSION

9/11

Mark was seen in the emergency room and admitted to the hospital. He was doing well until seven days ago, when he started running elevated temperatures and complaining of pains in the chest and back that were worse with deep inspiration. The chest and back pains subsided two to three days later and were followed with pains in the joints of the shoulders, elbows, and the right temporal mandibular areas. Mark's appetite has decreased. Diplopia was noted yesterday and transiently on the day of admission.

Mark did not appear to be in acute distress on admission. The physical exam was negative except for a slightly inflamed pharynx and mild tenderness in the right temporal mandibular joint. Mark's complete blood count showed a hemoglobin of 9.8 g percent, hematocrit of 32 percent, white blood count 1,600 and 37 percent segmenters, 44 percent lymphocytes, and adequate platelets. A lumbar spinal puncture revealed an increased cerebral spinal fluid pressure with 1 white blood cell, 970 red blood cells, 54 mg percent glucose, and 15 mg percent protein. Bone marrow aspiration was attempted on two different occasions and an adequate specimen for diagnosis was not obtained at either time. Cultures of the cerebral spinal fluid, the stool, the urine, the nose, and the throat were all negative. Three blood cultures grew out *Staphylococcus aureus* coagulase negative in various media. The chest x ray was normal. A liver scan revealed minimal hepatosplenomegaly. The brain scan was normal. A long bone survey was negative for infection or metastases. X rays of the temporal mandibular joints were normal.

Because of the initial blood cultures that revealed *Staphylococcus aureus* coagulase negative, Mark was treated with intravenous methicillin. Mark was febrile on admission and spiked temperatures to 40°C daily. Methicillin was started shortly after admission, and although there was some initial drop in the temperature (between 37.5° and 38°C) for the first two days of treatment, Mark's temperature was spiking up over

39°C after the initial drop. Because there had been no real improvement in Mark's febrile course in spite of adequate methicillin therapy and because the blood cultures revealed that the coagulase negative Staphylococci were also sensitive to aqueous penicillin, Mark was put on very high doses of intravenous aqueous penicillin. Three days after the penicillin had been started, there still was no change in Mark's clinical course. It was then decided that Mark might be in an exacerbation of his lymphocytic leukemia and that a trial on prednisone for 48 hours would be attempted and his temperature course watched closely. Mark was started on prednisone in the morning and that evening he was afebrile. He remained afebrile for three and a half days. The prednisone was tapered off, and it was felt that Mark was in an exacerbation because of his resopnse to prednisone. It was then decided that reinduction with Cytoxan therapy orally would be tried and that this could be done on an outpatient basis. Mark was discharged September 30 on 75 mg of Cytoxan orally daily to be followed in the clinic.

CLINIC VISITS

10/6

Mark is asymptomatic and currently is taking daily 75 mg of Cytoxan and 30 mg of prednisone. Mark's fever and bone pains respond very well to prednisone. It is felt at this time that the fever and bone pain are due to the disease process itself. There is no evidence of infection. The plan is to continue the prednisone and Cytoxan. Hemoglobin 9.8 g percent, hematocrit 29.2 percent, white blood count 3,200, segmenters 53 percent, lymphocytes 37 percent, and platelets 249,000.

10/20

Mark has been complaining of pain in his left thigh for one week. He has been taking codeine every six hours for the pain and the prednisone was increased to 60 mg daily three days ago. Since then the pain has decreased. Mark had a tender left thigh on physical exam. An x ray was taken. Plan to watch for two to three days. If there is no improvement, may consider giving radiation therapy to the left leg. Hemoglobin 10.3 g percent, white blood count 2,320, segmenters 62 percent, lymphocytes 31 percent, and platelets 54,000.

EMERGENCY ROOM VISITS

10/30

Mark was seen in the emergency room at 2:30 A.M. About two weeks ago Mark had sharp pains in his left thigh. At this time the prednisone was increased and the pain disappeared. He is currently in the emergency room due to pains in his right knee and lower abdomen, which began about 6:00 P.M. and have become increasingly worse since that time. The pain varies in intensity, is sharp in nature, and is only partially affected by position. His mother has been giving Empirin Compound #3 every three hours without benefit. Mark was given some intramuscular Demerol and sent home.

10/30
Mark returned to the emergency room about noon because of pain in his knee. The Demerol had given him relief through the night but the pain started again this morning. Mark is unable to extend his leg fully. There is no evidence of swelling or redness. A spinal tap was done with an opening pressure of 330 cm of water. Twelve mg of methotrexate was given intrathecally and 12 mg of citrovorum factor was given subcutaneously.

10/31
Mark came to the emergency room for intrathecal medication. A spinal tap was done with an opening pressure of 220 cm of water. Twelve mg of methotrexate was given intrathecally and 12 mg of citrovorum factor was given subcutaneously.

11/2
A radiotherapy consultation was done. It was felt that there was central nervous system leukemia with local involvement of the lumbosacral roots on the right. It was decided to start a course of cobalt therapy to the lumbosacral spine (four treatments in three days) beginning November 3 with 500 total rads.

FOURTH HOSPITAL ADMISSION

11/3
Mark was seen in the clinic complaining of severe bone pains in his right arm and leg. Demerol and codeine were not relieving his pain, and he was admitted to the hospital for control of pain with morphine.

On physical exam Mark presented a cushionoid appearance. Vital signs were normal. Eyes, ears, nose, and throat were within normal limits. The neck was supple. The lungs were clear to auxcultation. The abdomen was negative. Mark complained of extreme pain when his right arm was manipulated. His skin did not feel warm. His joints were not swollen and the pulses were good. There was tenderness over the right thigh when the knee was flexed. The neurological exam is within normal limits.

The urinalysis was unremarkable. Admission completed blood count showed a hemoglobin 8.5 g percent, white blood count 1,500 with 55 percent segmenters, 22 percent lymphocytes, and decreased platelets. The blood cultures revealed coagulase negative Staphylococci. The nose and throat cultures were unremarkable. The spinal fluid was negative. The chest x ray was normal. The bone marrow revealed an exacerbation of leukemia.

Mark was transfused with packed red cells, given vincristine intravenously and started on prednisone. Morphine was given for pain with no relief.

Although Mark had been told he had leukemia at the time of diagnosis, the nurse working with Mark felt that he was afraid of something which was related to the lack of morphine effectiveness. In talking with Mark, the nurse said, "I know you hurt but I think you hurt inside where the shots can't reach. I think you're afraid and I would be too." Mark did not respond verbally. Then the nurse asked, "Has anyone, like the doctors, nurses, or your friends, said anything to you to make you afraid?" Mark then relayed that a cousin had told him he was going to die. The nurse asked, "What do you think your cousin meant by that?" Mark did not know. The nurse continued, "As we have said, there isn't a cure for leukemia, just as there isn't a cure for diabetes [the nurse had discussed this before with Mark]. But this is why we give the medicines that are so strong and why they are given so often." Mark nodded his head. The nurse went on, "Mark, we don't know how or when any of us are going to die."

After this conversation with Mark, the nurse talked at length with Mark's mother about what had happened and Mark's response to what the nurse had said. The nurse told the mother that this response was normal and was to be expected. She also supported the mother telling her that Mark's response did not relate to anything she had done or failed to do. His reaction was normal and expected.

After talking with the mother, the nurse talked with Mark's doctor. He also talked to the mother and Mark. He took Mark to his office, re-explained leukemia, and had Mark look at slides under the microscope. Mark was told by the doctor at this time that anytime he was admitted and he felt that it was his last admission and asked the nurse or the doctors, they would tell him. From this point on in Mark's illness, his pain subsided and he was happy and outgoing. Mark was dismissed November 8, improved, to be followed in the clinic.

CLINIC VISITS

11/12

Mark started complaining of pain in his left elbow today. The second dose of vincristine was given intravenously. Prednisone was continued. Hemoglobin 13.8 g percent, hematocrit 38 percent, white blood count 3,300, segmenters 27 percent, and platelets 35,000.

11/18

Mark is much better although he began having pain in his right leg today. The third dose of vincristine was given intravenously. Prednisone was continued. Hemoglobin 12.2 g percent, hematocrit 38 percent, white blood count 1,350, segmenters 38 percent, lymphocytes 44 percent, and platelets 91,000.

11/23

Mark's right leg has continued to hurt. Last Sunday he had a headache. Last night his arms, legs, and back were quite uncomfortable, necessitating the use of Empirin Compound #3 three different times. There is not much improvement today. The fourth dose of vincristine was given intravenously. Prednisone was continued. A prescription was given for Empirin Compound #3 and chloral hydrate. Hemoglobin 11.3 percent, white blood count 1,600, and platelets 109,000.

12/1

Mark had a spinal tap done today. Opening pressure was 350 cm of water and closing pressure was 150 cm of water. 15 cc of spinal fluid was withdrawn. The cerebral spinal fluid showed 28 white blood cells and 80 percent mononuclears. It was decided to start a second course of cobalt radiation to the brain and cervical spine as a palliative measure. Seven treatments over a nine-day period with the total dose being 1,200 rads was begun (December 3 through 11). The fifth dose of vincristine was given intravenously. Prednisone was continued. Hemoglobin 8.7 g percent, white blood count 1,800, and platelets 28,000.

FIFTH HOSPITAL ADMISSION

12/5

Mark was admitted to the hospital for a blood transfusion and was transfused with two units of packed red blood cells. He tolerated the procedure well and at the time of discharge (December 6) he had a hemoglobin of 13.4 g percent and a hematocrit of 38.5 percent.

CLINIC VISITS

12/8

Mark is still receiving radiation therapy. White blood cells 600 and platelets 29,000. It was decided not to give vincristine.

12/11

Mark was seen in the emergency room complaining of nausea and malaise. There were no other symptoms. Radiation therapy was completed today and his headaches and extremity pain have disappeared. Hemoglobin 12.2 g percent, hematocrit 34 percent, white blood count 600, and platelets 29,000. No vincristine was given today.

12/15

Mark was seen in the clinic today. He has only had five doses of vincristine. It was not given today because of the blood count. Hemoglobin 9.3 g percent, hematocrit 27 percent, white blood count 311, and platelets 31,000.

12/21

Mark is doing very well and is asymptomatic. The sixth dose of vincristine was given intravenously. Hemoglobin 9.6 g percent, hematocrit 26 percent, white blood count 1,200, and platelets 39,000.

12/24

Mark was seen again in the emergency room. He has been complaining of right leg pain since yesterday and has a rather severe limp. He received the seventh dose of vincristine intravenously. One unit of packed cells was given.

SIXTH HOSPITAL ADMISSION

12/30

Mark was admitted for transfusion because of his anemia. He was transfused with two units of packed cells. Mark spiked a temperature of 40.4°C on the second day of his hospitalization. Blood cultures were negative. He was placed on intravenous methicillin for the remainder of his hospitalization and his temperature came down. Also on the second day of his hospitalization, Mark was noted to have tenderness over the left cheekbone. Mark was to have his eighth dose of vincristine during this hospitalization, but this was withheld because of his low white blood cell count. Mark was discharged on January 4 with a hemoglobin of 13.0 g percent, hematocrit of 37 percent, and white blood count of 250. Mark will be followed by a private dentist for the possibility of an abscess and will be seen in the clinic.

CLINIC VISITS

1/12/72

The private dentist diagnosed a tooth abscess and a root canal was performed, giving relief of pain. Currently he feels great. The eighth dose of vincristine was given intravenously. Prednisone was continued. Hemoglobin 11.0 g percent, hematocrit 31.2 percent, white blood count 1,900, platelets 21,000.

1/19

Mark did well until January 16, when he began to have some pain, which did not last long, in his left lower leg. Now he has discomfort in his left ankle and right arm. Plan to admit this week and discuss experimental regime. Hemoglobin 8.7 g percent, white blood count 1,200, segmenters 72 percent, lymphocytes 20 percent, platelets 39,000.

SEVENTH HOSPITAL ADMISSION

1/21

Mark was admitted because he now presents as resistant to the usual chemotherapeutic agents and is in need of a transfusion. Recently Mark complained of pain in the medial aspects of both ankles, but the pains are decreasing. He also felt tired and weak but maintained a good appetite. Mark has not had any fevers since his tooth abscess.

Mark presents as a markedly cushinoid and pale boy with marked alopecia in no acute distress. His physical exam was within normal limits except that his liver was palpable 1.5 cm below the right costal margin. The spleen was palpable 2 cm below the left costal margin. The complete blood count showed hemoglobin 7.2 g percent, hematocrit 20 percent, white blood count 550, segmenters 20 percent, lymphocytes 30 percent, platelets 24,000.

Because of Mark's resistance to the usual means of chemotherapy, he was started on an experimental drug according to protocol using L-asparaginase, vincristine, and prednisone in combination. Mark underwent five days of intravenous therapy with L-asparaginase, had one injection of vincristine, and was put on prednisone every six hours. Mark was discharged in good condition on the fifth hospital day and was to return to the hospital in five days for another course of L-asparaginase. Mark tolerated the chemotherapy well and responded well to the blood transfusions. At the time of discharge his hemoglobin was 14.8 g percent. A bone marrow biopsy was attempted in several different places but no specimen was obtained.

EIGHTH HOSPITAL ADMISSION

2/1

Mark was admitted for his second series of five daily injections of L-asparaginase, continuation of daily prednisone every six hours, and vincristine weekly. Mark has no complaints. The pains previously present in his extremities are now absent.

His physical exam was unchanged except for very mild tenderness over the liver edge, which was about 3 cm from the right costal margin. The complete blood count showed hemoglobin 12.4 g percent, hematocrit 35 percent, white blood count 540, segmenters 16 percent, lymphocytes 24 percent, platelets 8,000, and 40 percent immature and undifferentiated mononuclears.

Mark had an uneventful hospital stay, receiving five daily doses of L-asparaginase 6,600 units intravenously, one dose of vincristine intravenously, and prednisone daily. Mark was discharged February 5, to be readmitted five days from now for further treatment.

NINTH HOSPITAL ADMISSION

2/11

Mark was admitted for the third series of five daily injections of L-asparaginase, daily prednisone, and weekly vincristine. Mark's only complaints were related to tenderness in both lower legs with exercise which began a few days ago. He has had a steady weight gain since the start of his current chemotherapy. Currently he is on bowel sterilization program with the use of gentamicin, vancomycin, and nystatin.

The physical exam revealed normal fundi and tympanic membranes with the presence of slight blurring of the disc margins. The pharynx was clear except for a soft tissue hematoma on the right tonsillar fossa. There were several areas of hyperemia in the pharynx without exudate. The liver was palpable 8 cm below the right costal margin. There was a slightly tender liver edge. The spleen was not felt. Examination of the extremities revealed tenderness to firm palpation in both calves. The rest of the exam was within normal limits. The complete blood count showed hemoglobin 9.3 g percent, hematocrit 27 percent, white blood count 310, segmenters 15 percent, lymphocytes 30 percent, platelets 1,000, and 35 percent blast cells. Uric acid was 2.3 mg percent. Cerebral spinal fluid culture was negative. Cerebral spinal fluid cell count showed 4 white blood cells, 1 red blood cell, glucose 74 mg percent, chloride 117 meq. per liter, and protein 34 mg percent.

During Mark's hospital stay he received five daily injections of L-asparaginase, two injections of vincristine, and prednisone daily. Mark developed a febrile illness which apparently localized in his pharynx. Mark had a slight cough along with the pharyngitis. Shortly after the onset of the febrile illness, Mark developed headaches, and a spinal tap showed an opening pressure of 220 cm of water. Because of the high opening pressure, Mark was treated with one dose of intrathecal methotrexate and given citrovorum factor subcutaneously. Mark tolerated the spinal tap well and was covered prior to the spinal tap with platelet infusions. Mark was discharged in fairly good condition February 18, to be followed in the clinic.

TENTH HOSPITAL ADMISSION

2/20

Mark was seen in the emergency room complaining of abdominal pain and admitted to the hospital. The history was obtained from Mark's mother, who states that one day prior to discharge Mark began complaining of intermittent abdominal pain. The day prior to admission Mark complained of abdominal pain when he walked, urinated, or had a stool. Mrs. Davis also noticed some blood in the stool two days before admission but none since that time. The day of admission Mark began complaining of diffuse constant abdominal pain. His temperature the morning of admission was 39°C. No vomiting or diarrhea was noted.

The physical exam revealed a cushinoid white male in moderate distress. Conjunctival hemorrhages were seen bilaterally. Mark's abdomen appeared distended and bowel sounds were decreased. Mark's abdomen was tender in all quadrants. The skin showed multiple ecchymotic areas.

A flat plate of the abdomen was done on admission, which showed signs suggestive of ileus. Mark continued to complain of severe abdominal pain and was spiking a temperature. Because of this abdominal pain, valium intramuscularly was given. Over the next six hours Mark began to appear more stuporous and became quite agitated. He was given Demerol, gentamicin, and methicillin. Over the next four hours Mark showed marked deterioration of the sensorium and was pronounced dead on February 21 at 1:30 A.M.

STUDY GUIDE

1. What physiological alterations occur in leukemia with the erythrocytes, lymphocytes, and platelets? What nursing actions are indicated to assist the patient and family in preventing complications of the disease?
2. What is the basic disease process in leukemia? What effect does this have on the ability to withstand infection? What actions might be taken to help prevent infection?
3. Why is the bone marrow aspiration performed when leukemia is suspected?
4. What are the nursing responsibilities before and after a bone marrow aspiration is done?
5. What is the hematological picture of acute lymphocytic leukemia in exacerbation? Remission?
6. During Mark's illness, he received many medications. For each drug that he received,
   a. what is the drug classification?
   b. what is the expected physiological action?
   c. what are the side effects and toxic effects?
   d. what are the nursing implications?
7. What are the short- and long-term nursing care goals in working with a child with leukemia and his family in the different stages of the disease?
   a. diagnosis
   b. remission
   c. exacerbation
   d. terminal
   e. post death
8. Why is assessment of financial and insurance status of the family an important aspect of the total patient care? What resources are available to these families?
9. What are the normal developmental tasks for a boy nine years of age?
10. Discuss how the diagnosis of leukemia and the illness course might have influenced Mark's normal physical and psychosocial development.
11. Discuss how the parents perceive their child with a life-threatening illness. What impact does this have on their child-rearing practices? How might intra-family relationships be affected?
12. Are variables present in how the parents and child perceive a life-threatening illness? Discuss this.
13. How can religious beliefs help or hinder the child and family in coping with the disease process?

14. Discuss the commonalities in working with any family that has one of its members diagnosed with a fatal illness.

SELECTED READINGS

J. Q. Benoliel, "The Concept of Care for the Child with Leukemia," *Nursing Forum*, vol. XI, no. 2, 1972, pp. 194–204.

F. Bright and Sister L. Lance, "The Nurse and the Terminally Ill Child," *Nursing Outlook*, vol. 15, no. 9, September 1967, pp. 39–42.

B. Brodie, "The Nurse's Reaction to the Ill Child," *Nursing Clinics of North America*, vol. 1, no. 1, March 1966, pp. 95–101.

C. C. Congdon, "Bone Marrow Transplantation," *Science*, vol. 171, no. 3976, March 19, 1971, pp. 1116–1124.

C. Cragg, "The Child with Leukemia," *The Canadian Nurse*, vol. 65, no. 10, October 1969, pp. 30–34.

D. Galiardi and M. S. Miles, "Interactions Between Two Mothers of Children Suffering from Incurable Cancer," *Nursing Clinics of North America*, vol. 4, no. 1, March 1969, pp. 89–100.

D. P. Geis, "Mothers' Perceptions of Care Given Their Dying Children," *American Journal of Nursing*, vol. 65, no. 2, February 1965, pp. 105–107.

L. Goldfogel, "Working with the Parent of a Dying Child," *American Journal of Nursing*, vol. 70, no. 8, August 1970, pp. 1675–1679.

P. A. Holsclaw, "Nursing in High Emotional Risk Areas," *Nursing Forum*, vol. 4, no. 4, 1965, pp. 36–45.

W. T. Hughes, "Fatal Infections in Childhood Leukemia," *American Journal of Diseases of Children*, vol. 122, no. 4, October 1971, pp. 283–287.

M. Karon and J. Vernick, "An Approach to the Emotional Support of Fatally Ill Children," *Clinical Pediatrics*, vol. 7, no. 5, May 1968, pp. 274–280.

B. M. Livingston and I. H. Krafoff, "L-Asparaginase—A New Type of Anticancer Drug," *American Journal of Nursing*, vol. 70, no. 9, September 1970, pp. 1910–1915.

J. S. Lowenberg, "The Coping Behaviors of Fatally Ill Adolescents and Their Parents," *Nursing Forum*, vol. 9, no. 3, 1970, pp. 269–287.

J. N. Lukens and M. R. Miles, "Childhood Leukemia: Meeting the Needs of the Patient and Family," *Missouri Medicine*, vol. 67, no. 4, April 1970, pp. 224–236.

J. L. Lunceford, "Leukemia—Disease Process, Chemotherapeutic Approach and Nursing Care," *Nursing Clinics of North America*, vol. 2, no. 4, December 1967, pp. 635–647.

J. Q. Matthias, "Bone Marrow Biopsy," *Nursing Times*, vol. 67, no. 31, August 5, 1971, pp. 947–950.

A. M. Mauer, *Pediatric Hematology*, McGraw-Hill, New York, 1969, pp. 335–369.

T. M. Miya, "The Child's Perception of Death," *Nursing Forum*, vol, 11, no. 2, 1972, pp. 214–220.

D. A. Pacyna, "A Response to A Dying Child," *Nursing Clinics of North America*, vol. 5, no. 3, September 1970, pp. 421–430.

Progress Against Cancer 1969: A Report by the National Advisory Cancer Council. U.S. Department of Health, Education, and Welfare: Public Health Service, National Institutes of Health, National Cancer Institute.

E. K. Ross, "What Is It Like To Be Dying?" *American Journal of Nursing*, vol. 71, no. 1, January 1971, pp. 54–60.

J. E. Schowalter, "The Child's Reaction to His Own Terminal Illness," in Bernard Schoenberg *et al.* (eds.), *Loss and Grief: Psychological Management in Medical Practice*, Columbia University Press, New York, 1970.

A. A. Serpick, "Acute Versus Chronic Leukemia: Differential Features and Treatment," *Hospital Medicine*, vol. 6, no. 12, December 1970, pp. 7–21.

E. H. Waechter, "Children's Awareness of Fatal Illness," *American Journal of Nursing*, vol. 71, no. 6, June 1971, pp. 1168–1172.

Miss Blackwell

sixteen years old

Toxemia/Acute

Rosemary Cannon Kilker and Betty L. Wilkerson

Grace is a sixteen-year-old high school sophomore. She is an average student who hopes to complete high school and become a secretary.

Grace's father and mother have been divorced since she was a small child. Her mother is unemployed but is frequently away from home. Grace has five siblings, but only a nineteen-year-old sister remains at home.

Grace was brought to the maternity clinic by her sister, in whom she finally confided. She told her sister that the father of the baby is George, a classmate of the same age whom she had dated occasionally. George was the first person who had offered her any affection. The first menstrual period Grace missed, she passed off as being due to anemia. It was after the third period was missed that she informed George of the suspected pregnancy. Grace was hoping George would suggest eloping. Instead, he asked how he could be sure that the baby was his. Grace was shattered and was unable to function normally at home or at school. George stopped seeing Grace and totally ignored her on chance encounters.

In the clinic Grace was withdrawn, apprehensive, and extremely frightened. It was difficult for the physician to obtain any information. She cried out during the pelvic examination and afterward complained that the physician was deliberately hurting her. According to Grace, her mother's reaction to this pregnancy was anger and condemnation. Her mother told her that she was to stay at home, be cared for at the clinic, and that the baby was to be given up for adoption.

The mother made these plans without considering Grace's feelings.

THE INITIAL INTERVIEW AT THE CLINIC

At the first meeting of Grace and the clinic nurse, the nurse was unaware of her marital status. The conversation progressed as follows:

Nurse: "Hello, I'm Betty Brown. You are Grace Blackwell?"
Grace: "Yes."

Nurse: "Well, Grace, I'd like to ask you a few questions so I can start your health record. Are you married or single?"

Grace: "Single."

Nurse: "Are you about 16 or 17 years old?"

Grace: "16."

Nurse: "Do you remember the first day of your last normal menstrual period?"

Grace: "June 18." (squirming in her chair)

Nurse: "Any previous pregnancies?"

Grace: "No!" (angry)

Nurse: "How much did you weigh before you became pregnant?"

Grace: "106 pounds."

Betty Brown continued to ask questions to complete the opening of the health record. She ended the conversation by saying, "I think that's all the questions I have for the moment, Grace. Are there any questions I might answer for you?" When Grace shook her head, Miss Brown continued, "I will be with you during your visit today and will tell you what to expect before each procedure. Also, I will be with you at your subsequent visits."

NURSING ASSESSMENT AND ACTIVITIES

First Clinic Visit—Supportive Care

1. Rapport and communication
   a. Nursing history
      (1) Record
      (2) Kardex
   b. Evaluation of family situation and home environment
2. Preparation of record
3. Physical evaluation
   a. Blood pressure
   b. Fetal heart rate
   c. Weight
   d. Urine
   e. Papanicolaou smear preparation
   f. Assistance with examination
      (1) General physical evaluation
      (2) Obstetrical evaluation
4. Anticipatory guidance
   a. Importance of keeping antepartal appointments
   b. Antepartum instructions
   c. Interpretation of physician's orders
5. Need for referral to social services and dietary

The physician's examination, January 29, 1968, revealed a well-developed, well-nourished female with estimated date of confinement March 25, 1968; a uterine gestation of 32-week size, fetal heart rate 140, blood pressure 130/90, and no visible edema. Her weight gain was 13.61 kg. Grace was advised to reduce her caloric and salt intake and scheduled to return to the clinic in one week. A conference with the social worker and dietician was arranged by the nurse.

In this clinic, the following laboratory tests and examinations are done:

Complete history and physical
Urinalysis at each visit
Blood pressure at each visit
Serology
Complete blood count
Rh factor
Blood typing
Cervical smear
Papanicolaou smear
F.H.T.

Grace's second clinic visit was not kept. She did not return to the clinic until three weeks later.

Second Clinic Visit—Supportive Care
(Three Weeks Late)

1. Continuation of rapport and communication
   a. Psychological needs
   b. Dietary needs
   c. Physical needs
2. Anticipatory guidance
   a. Reinforcement of physician's orders
   b. Importance of keeping antepartal appointments
   c. Telephone call
   d. Home visit
3. Physical evaluation
   a. General assessment
   b. Urine
   c. Blood pressure
   d. Fetal heart rate
   e. Weight
   f. Fundal measurement

At this time, Grace's blood pressure was 144/96. She had a weight gain of 1.81 kg, proteinuria 1+, fetal heart rate 138, and minimal edema of hands and feet. A tentative diagnosis of mild preeclampsia was made. Grace was instructed regarding a 1,500-mg sodium diet and advised to obtain extra rest and to return to the clinic in one week.

Betty Brown took Grace to a quiet area and discussed with Grace the doctor's diagnosis of preeclampsia. Miss Brown said, "Grace, I want to help you. What can I do?" Grace responded, "The whole thing . . . I'm just sick of the whole business. That diet jazz is way out." This gave Betty an opening to go over the diet step by step and to help her plan her meals and snacks. After this discussion Miss Brown said, "Now Grace, we *can* count on you being back in one week, can't we?" Grace answered, "Oh yeah, I'll come."

Grace did keep her next appointment and arrived at the clinic one week later. She had a 0.91-kg weight gain. However, her other tests remained the same. She was placed on Hygroten 100 mg every other day and was to continue her diet and rest and to return to the clinic in four days.

Third Clinic Visit—Supportive Care

1. Continuation of previous listed nursing interventions
2. Explanation of medication
3. Talk of possible hospitalization
4. Emphasizing the need to return in four days

Miss Brown praised Grace for returning to the clinic as requested. Grace asked the nurse, "How sick am I?" Miss Brown replied, "Grace, you are a sick girl. That is why you must rest, take the medication the doctor has prescribed every other day, and stay on that diet. If your condition doesn't improve, you will have to be hospitalized to lower your blood pressure and help you to feel better." Grace said, "Oh yes, I really don't feel good. You'll see me in four days. You'll be here again, won't you?"

When Grace arrived in the clinic four days later, her blood pressure was 148/105, her weight loss was 0.45 kg. However, the proteinuria remained at 1+. The physician decided to admit her to the hospital for observation and treatment.

Fourth Clinic Visit and Admission to Hospital— Supportive Care

1. Clinic evaluation
2. Preparation for admission to hospital
3. Assistance with admission procedures

After the physician left the room, Grace turned to Miss Brown and began to cry. "I don't feel good. I am getting worse." The nurse put her arm around Grace and said, "I understand that you don't feel good, and being in the hospital a few days will help you to feel better. Does your mom know you haven't been feeling well? Did she or your sister come with you today?" Grace responded, "My sister's here again. You know my mother never comes."

Miss Brown explained some of the admission procedures and took Grace, accompanied by her sister, to the maternity unit.

Upon admission to the hospital on March 8, 1968, Grace's blood pressure was 148/105, pulse 100/minute, respiration 16/minute, and fetal heart rate 144. The physician's findings stated that the eye grounds were benign. There was moderate edema of the eyelids, hands, and ankles, and some blurring of vision. The neurological exam was essentially negative. The estimated gestation was 37 weeks, and the estimated fetal weight was 2.50 kg. Vaginal examination revealed an unengaged vertex presentation, 1 cm dilatation, and 50 percent effacement of cervix and intact membranes.

The diagnosis of the attending physician was preeclampsia. The following orders were written:

1. Bed rest
2. Intake and output
3. Weight daily
4. 24 hr urine for protein
5. Blood pressure q. 4 h.
6. Phenobarbitol 30 mg q.i.d. orally
7. Seconal 100 mg H.S. orally
8. 1,500 mg Na, 1,500 calorie diet
9. Blood chemistry
10. Fetal age (x ray)
11. Hygroten 100 mg q. other day
12. Eclamptic precautions

Admission and First Day of Acute Care

1. Admission procedures
   a. Selection of proper environment
   b. Temperature, pulse, respiration
   c. Fetal heart rate, blood pressure
   d. Weight
   e. Collecting admission urine
   f. Nursing evaluation of patient's needs
   g. Assisting patient's adaptation to environment

    h.   Explanation of hospital routine in regard to her care

    i.   Toxemia tray at bedside

2. Personal care

    a.   Bed bath if feasible

    b.   Controlled environment

        (1) Planned period of rest

        (2) Planned period of nursing activities

            (a)   Check elimination

            (b)   Give medications as ordered on time

            (c)   Assist with lab tests

            (d)   Close observation of patient's intake and output

            (e)   Observe for signs of labor

            (f)   Observe for signs of complications: dizziness, headache, epigastric pain

            (g)   Coordinate activities with paramedical team members

    c.   Interpret patient's care to the patient and family

Twenty-four hours following admission Grace complained of frontal headache, blurring of vision, and had obvious facial and hand edema. Her blood pressure was 148/110, and fetal heart rate was 138. During this same period her intake was 2,400 cc and her output was 1,250 cc. The twenty-four hour urine protein revealed 1 g of protein. She demonstrated hyperreflexia. The BUN was 30 mg percent. The fetal film revealed no distal femoral epiphysis. The estimated fetal weight was given at 2.50 kg. It was felt that with the above findings, Mg SO$_4$ and morphine were the drugs of choice at this time.

Toxemia Tray

Magnesium sulfate, 50%
Calcium gluconate
Syringes—needles—tourniquet, pledgets
Padded tongue blade
Stimulants
Sedatives
Reflex hammer
50 cc 50% glucose

Physician's Orders

1. N.P.O.

2. 1,000 cc 5% glucose/water I.V. run in 8 hr, followed by another 1,000 cc of 5% glucose Ringer's in the next 12 hr

3. Mg SO₄, 10 g, 50% solution deep I.M., to be followed by 5 g every 6 hr deep I.M., 1 procaine may be used
4. Morphine, 10 mg, to be administered I.M. stat and q. 8 h.
5. Foley catheter
6. Weight daily
7. I & O
8. Repeat fetal x ray
9. Blood pressure q. 1 h.

Second Day of Acute Care

1. Continuation of previous nursing activities
   a. Blood pressure q. 1 h.
   b. Side rails padded in anticipation of convulsions
   c. Close observation for signs of labor when medicated with
      (1) Magnesium sulfate
      (2) Morphine
   d. Check knee jerk, respirations, and urine output
   e. Regulation and notation of intravenous therapy
   f. Constant observation of patient
2. Further interpretation to family of patient's condition

On the third day of hospitalization, fetal heart rate was 140, blood pressure was 140/100, and Grace had a 1.36-kg weight loss.

Physician's Orders

1. Repeat fetal x ray
2. Amniocentesis for fetal age
3. Continue preeclamptic regime

Third Day of Acute Care

1. Continuation of previous nursing care
2. Explaining amniocentesis to Grace and family

The fetal x ray revealed continued doubtful age of the fetus. The amniotic fluid was tested for determining fetal age. Fetal age at this time was estimated at 36 weeks. The 24-hour urine protein was 0.8 g. Grace's reflexes were slightly irritable and her eye grounds were negative. Her temperature was normal and her intake was 2,800 cc with an output of 3,500 cc.

Around 3 A.M. the next morning, Grace was observed to be having periodic intervals of restlessness. Contractions were timed as occurring every four to five minutes with a duration of 30 seconds and of fair quality.

Upon vaginal examination, her cervix was 1 cm dilated, 80% effaced and with the vertex presenting at a minus 1 station. At 4:30 A.M. another vaginal examination revealed the cervix to be 2 to 3 cm dilated and 80% effaced with the presenting part at 0 station. Grace was having contractions every 2 to 3 minutes, of 35 to 40 seconds duration and of fairly good quality. Her blood pressure was 138/100 and fetal heart rate 152.

Fourth Day of Acute Care

In the Labor Area

1. Transfer to labor area
2. Admission procedure with perineal prep
3. Constant attendance
   a. Time contractions
   b. Fetal heart rate and blood pressure every 15 minutes
   c. Reassure her of her progress
   d. Vaginal examinations to determine progress
   e. Relieve back pain with pressure of hands
   f. Continue previous nursing activities
4. Interpretation of patient's progress to family

As labor progressed toward termination, Grace aroused with her contractions and complained of severe backache saying, "My back is killing me." An epidural anesthetic was given for analgesia. Due to Grace's condition, she was transferred to the delivery room at this time.

Five hours, eight minutes after labor commenced, a live born male infant was delivered by low forceps over a midline episiotomy. Following Grace's delivery, *the physician wrote the following orders:*

1. Record I & O
2. V.S. q. 15 min x4, then q. 30 min x4, then q. 2 h. while awake
3. Tox precautions
4. Regular diet
5. Ambulate in 8 hr
6. Tucks to perineum
7. Milk of magnesia 30 cc P.O. p.r.n. constipation
8. Catheterize if unable to void in 8 hr
9. Darvon compound 65 mg every 4 hr p.r.n. for pain
10. Hgb. and hematocrit 2nd postpartum day

In the Maternity Recovery Room. Immediate postpartum care included:

1. Continue eclamptic precautions
2. Administer oxytoxic preparation
3. Palpate fundus
4. Determine amount of vaginal flow
5. Cleanse vulva
6. Check vital signs every 15 minutes
7. Remain in intensive care for approximately 24 hr

Immediately postpartum Grace's blood pressure was 130/96, pulse 88, fundus was firm, and she had a minimum amount of bleeding. The intravenous fluids were discontinued when completed.

Convalescent Postpartum Care

1. Do daily 8-point check
2. Weigh daily
3. Begin patient caring for self
4. Provide opportunity for birth control discussion
5. Encourage patient to return for six-week checkup
6. Interpret postpartum danger signs
7. Demonstrate postpartum exercises
8. Advise as to early medical attention in future pregnancy

Grace's blood pressure decreased to 120/90 the day following delivery. On her first and second postpartum days, her total body diuresis was estimated at 3,000 cc per day. She was free of headache, proteinuria, and edema. Weight loss was 6.75 kg.

The hospital social worker visited Grace daily and verified that she wished to relinquish the baby. Final arrangements were made with the adoption agency. The postpartum period was uneventful and Grace was discharged in four days to return to the clinic in two weeks. Discharge instructions included a discussion of the use of contraceptives, diet control, and social adjustment.

Eight-point Check of the Postpartum Mother

1. Breasts
2. Uterus
3. Lochia
4. Bladder
5. Episiotomy
6. Bowel movement

7. Homan's sign
8. Emotional stage

THE BABY

The cord was around the neck two times and the Apgar score was 5, one minute post delivery. Five minutes following delivery, the Apgar was 8. Birth weight of this infant was 1.71 kg. The baby was placed in an isolette for nine days. As the baby's suck reflex was poor, a nasal gastric tube was in place for the first seven days. The baby's growth and development was uneventful. At the end of four weeks his weight was 2.5 kg. and he was dismissed to the adoption agency.

STUDY GUIDE

1. What factors enter into the development of a sixteen-year-old's personality structure?
2. What identifications are necessary for a sixteen-year-old girl?
3. What effect does pregnancy have on the circulatory system? Would there be a variance between the adolescent and the adult?
4. What are the nutritional needs of an expectant mother? Does adolescence alter these needs?
5. Will an adolescent have more complications during pregnancy, labor, and delivery than a mature woman?
6. What cues can you pick up from the interview that would help the nurse build a relationship with Grace?
7. How could the nurse have supported the physician while also supporting Grace at the time of the initial examination?
8. How does preeclampsia differ from eclampsia?
9. What are some of the factors that are thought to predispose to toxemia?
10. In the diagnosis of true toxemia it must be distinguished from what other medical conditions?
11. What ongoing nursing assessments can be made to facilitate early diagnosing of toxemia and to differentiate toxemia from other conditions?
12. What are the possible complications of toxemia of pregnancy?
13. Why is the infant of a mother with toxemia classified as "high risk?"
14. What are the significant blood chemistry values in the toxemia patient?
15. Compare the physiological changes that occur in toxemia with those of normal pregnancy.
16. Why use magnesium sulfate in the twentieth century?
17. What knowledge and precautions are necessary before administering magnesium sulfate?

18. Why are diuretics used?
19. What are the prodromal signs and symptoms of eclampsia?
20. What nursing assessments and nursing care need to be ongoing to assist in preventing eclampsia?
21. In regard to the unwed mother:
    a. How can the nurse go about helping this unwed girl?
    b. Would you feel differently toward an unwed girl if she were sixteen rather than twenty-eight?
    c. What is the nurse's role in advising the mother whether to keep the baby or place it for adoption?
    d. Does the nurse have a responsibility to discuss sexual activity and birth control with Grace?
22. How do you see the nurse's role in each of the following areas?
    a. Antepartal clinic
    b. Antepartal nursing unit
    c. Labor and delivery
    d. Postpartal nursing unit
23. What type of labor is seen most frequently in the toxemic patient?

SELECTED READINGS

H. M. Adams and Y. Gallaghu, "Some Facts and Observations about Illegitimacy," *Children*, March–April 1963, p. 43.

V. Apgar *et al.*, "Evaluation of the Newborn Infant—Second Report," *Journal of the American Medical Association*, December 13, 1958.

F. Coffina, "Helping a Mother Surrender Her Child for Adoption," *Child Welfare*, February 1960, p. 25.

J. F. Donnelly, "Toxemia of Pregnancy," *American Journal of Nursing*, April 1961, pp. 98–101.

E. Fitzpatrick *et al.*, *Maternity Nursing*, 12th ed., J. B. Lippincott, Philadelphia, 1971, pp. 448–458.

C. E. Flowers, "Magnesium Sulfate in Obstetrics," *American Journal of OB and GYN*, March 15, 1965, pp. 763–776.

A. Grollman, "Diuretics," *American Journal of Nursing*, January 1965, pp. 84–89.

L. M. Hellman and J. Pritchard, *Williams Obstetrics*, 14th ed., Appleton-Century-Crofts, New York, 1971, pp. 685–739.

C. H. Hendricks and W. Brenner, "Toxemia of Pregnancy: Relationship Between Fetal Weight, Fetal Survival, and the Maternal State," *American Journal of OB and GYN*, January 15, 1971, pp. 231–233.

B. Highley, "Antepartal Nursing Intervention," *Nursing Forum*, no. 4, 1963, p. 62.

C. Hogue and M. Couch, "Care of the Patient with Toxemia," *American Journal of Nursing*, April 1961, pp. 101–103.

S. Israel and T. Wonteriz, "Teenage Obstetrics: A Cooperative Study," *American Journal of OB and GYN*, March 1, 1963, p. 659.

J. G. Loesch and N. Greenberg, "Some Specific Areas of Conflict Observed during Pregnancy: A Comparative Study of Married and Unmarried Pregnant Women," *American Journal of Orthopsychiatry*, July 1962, p. 624.

M. MacLaverty *et al.*, "Program for Toxemia Control," *American Journal of OB and GYN*, May 1, 1965, pp. 100–105.

National Academy of Science, Committee on Maternal Nutrition/Food and Nutrition: *Maternal Nutrition and the Course of Pregnancy: Summary Report*, Washington, D.C.

National Dairy Council, "Teenage Nutrition," *Dairy Council Digest*, January–February 1964.

F. Ostapowicz and O. Cavanaugh, "Management and Prevention of Eclamptogenic Toxemia," *Hospital Topics*, September 1971, pp. 73–75.

O. Stine *et al.*, "Pregnancy in Adolescence," *Briefs*, April 1964, p. 58.

Mr. Sommers
twenty years old

Head Injury and Fractured Femur/Acute
Jeanne Quesenbury and Sara Hammes

Mr. Sommers, a twenty-year-old, lived in a small town in Missouri with his parents, brothers, and sisters. He worked as an auto mechanic and was in good health until December 6, 1969. On that date, he was on his way to a National Guard Meeting when his car crashed, shearing a telephone pole and throwing him from the car.

When Mr. Sommers was picked up about one hour later, he was taken to a small, nearby hospital. There a tracheostomy was performed and intravenous fluid administered. A right chest tube was inserted because x rays showed a minimal right pneumothorax. X rays also indicated that there was a right orbital fracture and a fracture of the left femur. He was then transferred to a medical center, where he remained for one month.

FIRST HOSPITAL DAY—DECEMBER 6

At 11:30 A.M. Mr. Sommers was admitted to the emergency room on a stretcher. He was semicomatose and restless. The right pupil was 7 mm in diameter and nonreactive; the left was 3 mm in diameter and reactive. There was bilateral periorbital edema and ecchymosis. The ear canals were clear. There was movement in all extremities, but less movement on the left side. Babinski signs were present bilaterally. His neck was supple. His chest had good breath sounds bilaterally and no rales were heard; the tracheostomy tube was in place and patent. The medical diagnosis at this time was as follows: severe cerebral contusion; rule out intracerebral or subdural hematoma. (A later and final diagnosis was: severe cerebral contusion with probable brain stem injury; blunt trauma to both globes, with associated choroidal rupture and vitreous hemorrhage; fracture of left femur.)

Other tests at the time of admission to the emergency room included a urinalysis, which was normal; complete blood count with the hemoglobin

14.3 g, hematocrit 41.7%, platelet count adequate, and white blood count 27,000. The blood gas studies showed a PO_2 of 47 and a PCO_2 of 34, giving a pH of 7.46. Electrolytes were as follows: sodium 144, potassium 3.6, and chloride 102. A carotid arteriogram by direct puncture was performed: there was good cross filling with no evidence of vessel displacement. X rays showed multiple facial fractures, the most pronounced being the right orbital fracture of the frontal region. The comminuted mid-shaft fracture of the left femur was also verified. Mr. Sommers was placed in skeletal traction for conservative management of his femur.

At 2 P.M. Mr. Sommers was admitted to the nursing unit on an x ray cart. Restraints were used because of his restlessness and because he moved all extremities with strength. Paraldehyde 5 cc was given intravenously. A Jelco catheter was inserted into the right femoral artery for purposes of measuring the arterial pressure and for arterial blood gas sampling; a catheter was placed into the right ankle vein for continuous intravenous fluid therapy; a cerebral spinal line was inserted into the subarachnoid space in the lumbar region and a silastic catheter was inserted, via cut-down, into the pulmonary artery for continuous central venous pressure monitoring and venous gas sampling. A lead II electrocardiogram was strapped to his right arm and to both legs for heart rate and electrocardiogram monitoring.

Physician's orders at this time were as follows:

1. Admit to Neurosurgery. Diagnosis: head injury with fractured femur and right pneumothorax. Condition: poor.
2. C.B.C., U.A., type and cross match for four units of whole blood.
3. Head trauma unit studies.
4. Vital signs and neuro signs every 1 hr.
5. Position in traction for Orthopedic Rx.
6. Intake and output with hourly output recorded. Fluid in the arterial catheter of 1,000 cc normal saline to run in 24 hr. Follow with 1,000 cc normal saline to run in 12 hr. and 1,000 cc 5% dextrose in water to run in 12 hr.
7. Ampicillin Gram 1, I.V. by volutrol every 6 hr.
8. Tetanus toxoid 0.5 cc I.M.
9. C.B.C., electrolytes in A.M.
10. Foley to dependent drainage.
11. Tracheostomy care.
12. Culture tracheal secretions and urine today.
13. Thorazine 50 mg I.M. for restlessness.

FIRST HOSPITAL WEEK—DECEMBER 7–14

Mr. Sommers's condition remained critical during the first few days. His nursing care included life-sustaining activities as well as precautionary measures that would benefit his rehabilitation. Oxygen was provided by means of the Bennett respirator, and its concentration was regulated by periodic blood gas studies. The respiratory equipment was checked to make sure that both oxygen and humidity were being supplied in correct amounts. Frequent tracheal and oral suctioning was required. For the latter procedure, sterile gloves and a new sterile catheter were employed each time that Mr. Sommers was suctioned. The skin around the tracheostomy was cleansed and the tracheostomy dressing was changed when necessary.

Mr. Sommers's level of consciousness and neurological status were observed hourly. The level of consciousness was ascertained by first of all calling Mr. Sommers by his given name, using a normal tone of voice. When there was no response a louder tone together with slight shaking movements to his body were used in the attempt to arouse him, and when he still did not respond, the skin over body prominences was pinched or pressed, with moderately painful stimuli or stronger pain stimulation. Mr. Sommers was observed to respond to moderately painful stimuli. This response to pain, together with the fact that frequently during the first few days Mr. Sommers was restless to the point of requiring Thorazine 50 mg intramuscularly or intravenously and restraints as precautionary safety measures, indicated that Mr. Sommers was at one of the intermediate levels of consciousness. He was, however, unable to grasp the nurse's hand or make other types of voluntary movements upon instruction. His pupils were checked by using the flashlight to observe whether both were equal in size and whether each separately responded to light and how quickly each responded. During the first part of this week, Mr. Sommers's right pupil remained dilated and fixed; the left was smaller and reactive. Changes in temperature, blood pressure, pulse, and respiration were looked for because of their relationship to increasing intracranial pressure and bleeding. Dilatin 300 mg was administered to Mr. Sommers daily, starting December 10.

He was incontinent of urine and feces, and it was necessary to use an indwelling catheter and observe the frequency of his bowel movements. The urinary drainage system used was of the closed sterile type, and collection of urine samples and bladder irrigations was accomplished with a sterile needle and syringe. The catheter was cleansed immediately below the retention tube and the needle inserted for the collection or irrigation procedure. The urethral meatus was cleansed as necessary, but at least twice a day.

Because Mr. Sommers's eyes remained closed, the danger of corneal ulceration was lessened somewhat. Normal saline was used to cleanse his eyes and eye drops moistened them. Oral hygiene was required and water-soluble lubricant helped his lips from becoming dry and cracked.

The traction for the fractured femur was observed for correct alignment and for an adequate amount of weight to provide for balance, suspension, traction, and countertraction. It was necessary to change the bed linens from the top of the bed to the bottom rather than from side to side, in order to maintain correct alignment of fractured bone. The skin area at the site of insertion of the Steinman pin was cleansed twice daily with pHisoHex and, because pHisoHex may be irritating to the skin, a sterile water cleansing to the skin followed.

Thorazine was unnecessary after the middle of the first week. The chest tube was removed and Mr. Sommers had no further respiratory problems. The central venous pressure monitoring was also discontinued. Unexplained bleeding through the urinary catheter was noticed toward the end of the first week, and it lasted for four days. His hemoglobin went down and he received transfusions with whole blood and packed cells. His electrolytes remained normal, as did the specific gravity.

SECOND HOSPITAL WEEK—DECEMBER 15–21

At the beginning of the second week, Mr. Sommers became very quiet. Decerebrate posturing was observed. During this week, his blood pressure was high and unstable, ranging from 185/90 to 200/120 mm Hg. Temperatures of 39.5°C and 40°C rectally occurred, with periods of diaphoresis. The blood, urine, spinal fluid, and tracheal secretions were cultured, but these showed negative growth at both twelve- and twenty-four-hour intervals. (The tracheostomy stoma was noted to have had a slight pseudomonous-type odor on one occasion.) Ampicillin Gram 1 every six hours, ordered on the date of admission, was discontinued on December 16 and kanamycin 500 mg intramuscularly every eight hours was started. Mr. Sommers became afebrile approximately two weeks after hospitalization and antibiotics were discontinued.

His conscious level appeared to be about the same: He responded to moderately painful stimuli but otherwise could not be roused. However, he did yawn and cough, and was able to cough up some of the secretions even though he still required frequent suctioning. The nurse's notes indicated that cup clapping loosened secretions considerably. He attempted to "breathe against the machine," and IPPB therapy was reduced and treatments were scheduled for 10 minutes out of each hour with no Bennett therapy during the remainder of each hour. When the Bennett was applied, the tracheostomy cuff was inflated; it remained deflated when the machine was not in use. On December 15, Ritalin 100 mg was started and was given every four hours.

Toward the end of the second week an order was written for Mr. Sommers to be sat up in bed b.i.d. A nasogastric feeding tube was passed with intake to be progressed to 240 cc of natural tube feeding and 80 cc of water every two hours. The medications were changed to P.O. at this time. Occasionally the tube feedings were omitted, either because of green-tinged material which was suctioned from the tracheostomy or because of large amounts of fluid which were aspirated from the stomach.

X rays of the femur at this time showed the fractured bone to be in good position; a calcified distal femur was visualized.

Mr. Sommers's mother was with her son frequently. Because she is a practical nurse, the hospital routine and many of the necessary procedures were not new to her. On the other hand, an astute nurse could easily detect her sadness at seeing her son so helpless and her fear about his uncertain future. Whenever it was appropriate, the mother was permitted to assist with the care of her son. For example, when Mr. Sommers began to tolerate his tube feedings better, she received instruction on their administration and fed him some of the time.

THIRD AND FOURTH HOSPITAL WEEK— DECEMBER 22–JANUARY 6

Mr. Sommers received Colace 100 mg three times daily per nasogastric tube. He required cleansing enemas on several occasions.

He now began to follow the movements of people near the head of his bed with his eyes, and occasionally he responded to basic verbal commands, such as "squeeze my hand." His blood pressure gradually stabilized. Follow-up x rays of the femur showed a mild degree of shortening and a slight lateral displacement of the distal fragment. On December 30, a left hip spica was applied.

On January 2, Mr. Sommers was moved onto a cart and wheeled into the hall. There he seemed to follow people with his eyes, turn his head toward voices at the nursing station, and move his hands in response to greetings.

On January 3, he pulled out the nasogastric tube. Attempts were made to offer him small amounts of water and he did swallow some of it. Once, however, he coughed severely and some of the water returned around the tracheostomy. It was therefore necessary for the feeding tube to be reinserted.

To assist with the hospital and medical costs, Mr. Sommers's mother applied for disability aid under the Social Security Act. And because the accident occurred when Mr. Sommers was enroute to a National Guard Meeting, financial assistance through the Veterans Administration was also applied for and received. Accordingly, post-hospital arrangements for extended and rehabilitative care at a Veterans Administration hospital were made.

On January 6, Mr. Sommers was transferred to that institution in an ambulance.

ADDENDUM

Mr. Sommers visited the nursing unit in early 1971. His mother brought him to the ward since he had an appointment in the orthopedic clinic. He used a cane for assistance in walking. He had no memory of the accident, his hospitalization here, or part of his hospitalization at the Veterans Administration hospital. (He had been at the Veterans Administration hospital for several months.) He was mentally alert and his mother thought that he was doing quite well. The head nurse had the impression that Mr. Sommers wanted to be more independent than his mother was allowing. It is unknown whether he was gainfully employed at this time.

STUDY GUIDE

Nursing Responsibilities Inherent in the Care of the Unconscious Patient

1. What pathological processes occurred inside the skull immediately following Mr. Sommers's injury?
2. What are "neurological signs?"
3. What is meant by the term "level of consciousness?"
4. How are the cause(s) and extent of head injury determined? That is, what diagnostic tests and neurological signs are used?
5. Of what significance are changes in neurological signs?
6. Discuss some of the ways you would try to obtain response from the unresponsive patient if he were at a level of consciousness similar to Mr. Sommers's. Why is such action necessary?

Areas of Care Associated with Head Injuries

Study the following areas of care associated with the patient who has a head injury.

1. Oxygen need: suction, tracheostomy care, cup clapping, the Bennett respirator, blood gas studies.
2. Fluids and nutrition: intravenous fluid therapy, tube feedings, precautions in giving tube feedings, oral hygiene.
3. Temperature and infection control: antibiotics, methods for providing hypothermia, catheter care.
4. Restlessness: medication, restraints.
5. Lethargy: medication, sensory stimulation (visual, auditory, tactile).
6. Pain: Does Mr. Sommers have an awareness of pain?
7. Disuse phenomenon: range of motion, skin care, eye care.
8. Complications of a head injury or fracture: respiratory acidosis, fat emboli, thrombi, pneumonia, gastrointestinal ulceration.
9. The family: How would you help Mr. Sommers's mother?

Nursing Responsibilities of the Patient in Traction and Casts

1. Skeletal traction
2. Balanced traction
3. Restricted movement
4. Prevention of infection
5. Maintenance of effective traction
6. Cast care

SELECTED READINGS

J. A. Bailey, "Balanced Traction-Suspension for a Fractured Femur in a Thrashing Patient," *Clinical Orthopaedics and Related Research*, vol. 51, March–April 1967, pp. 123–125.

J. A. Bailey, "Tractions, Suspensions and a Ringless Splint," *American Journal of Nursing*, vol. 70, August 1970, pp. 1724–1725.

C. Betson, "Blood Gases," *American Journal of Nursing*, vol. 68, May 1968, pp. 1010–1012.

A. P. Bray and J. Thomas, "Severe Fat Embolism Syndrome," *Nursing Times*, vol. 65, January 23, 1969, pp. 109–110.

E. Carini and G. Owens, *Neurological and Neurosurgical Nursing*, 5th ed., C. V. Mosby, St. Louis, 1970, pp. 270–278.

D. Carnevali and S. Brueckner, "Immobilization—Reassessment of a Concept," *American Journal of Nursing*, vol. 70, July 1970, pp. 1502–1507.

R. Davenport, "Tube Feeding for Long-Term Patients," *American Journal of Nursing*, vol. 64, January 1964, pp. 121–123.

R. N. De Jong, *The Neurological Examination*, 3rd ed., Harper & Row, New York, 1967, pp. 949–986.

J. R. Feild, "Head Injuries Patho-Physiology," *The Journal of the Arkansas Medical Society*, vol. 66, March 1970, pp. 340–347.

M. A. M. Gardner, "Responsiveness as a Measure of Consciousness," *American Journal of Nursing*, vol. 68, May 1968, pp. 1034–1038.

J. R. Green (ed.), "Seminar on the Management of Head Injuries," *Arizona Medicine*, vol. 25, February 1968, entire edition.

R. Hooper, *Patterns of Acute Head Injury*, Williams and Wilkins, Baltimore, 1969, pp. 109–129.

F. E. Jackson, "The Pathophysiology of Head Injuries," *Clinical Symposia*, vol. 18, no. 3, 1966.

F. E. Jackson, "The Treatment of Head Injuries," *Clinical Symposia*, vol. 19, no. 1, 1967.

C. B. Larson and M. Gould, *Orthopedic Nursing*, 7th ed., C. V. Mosby, St. Louis, 1970, pp. 37–84.

M. E. Leavens, "Brain Tumors," *American Journal of Nursing*, vol. 64, March 1964, pp. 78–81.

F. Plum, "Axioms on Coma," *Hospital Medicine*, vol. 4, May 1968, pp. 20–31.

J. Quesenbury and P. Lambright, "Observations and Care for Patients with Head Injuries," *The Nursing Clinics of North America*, vol. 4, June 1969, pp. 237–247.

H. A. Rusk (ed.), *Rehabilitation Medicine*, 3rd ed., C. V. Mosby, St. Louis, 1971, pp. 223–237, 448–462.

J. Secor, *Patient Care in Respiratory Problems*, W. B. Saunders, Philadelphia, 1969.

J. E. Thomas and G. D. Molnar, "The Unconscious Patient," *Hospital Medicine*, vol. 1, November 1968, pp. 6–22.

S. Thomas, "Fat Embolism—A Hazard of Trauma," *Nursing Times*, vol. 65, January 23, 1969, pp. 105–108.

Mr. Charles

twenty-one years old

Schizophrenia/Chronic

Loren O. King

Mr. Charles is a twenty-one-year-old, single male. He is 5 feet, 6 inches tall and weighs approximately 7.3 kg. He has two older sisters (four and six years older), who are married and have families of their own. He is the only son in the family. His mother is the only person living at home.

Mr. Charles's father was divorced from his mother when the patient was in preadolescence. The father died about two years later of pulmonary carcinoma. Not much is known about the father. According to the patient, he was an "alcoholic." The father seems to have been dominated by the mother, and also seems to have been a poor father figure and male role model for the patient.

Before his death and in periods of employment, the father worked as a butcher, and the mother told him which jobs to take. She also seems to have handled much of the family's finances. Mr. Charles relates: "My father would come home drunk and then my mother would tell him to leave home and not come back until he was sober." Apparently the father would comply, although not much doubt exists that this was a repetitive phenomenon.

Some idea of the quality of the father–son interaction is found in what happened when Mr. Charles went to his father with very basic questions about the "facts of life." His father would usually laughingly counter with some statement such as, "All you have to know is to always take rubbers along on a date in case you need them," or "If you want a good piece, don't pick someone like your old lady."

When Mr. Charles talked about his father, he never once gave any kind of suggestion that he had any memories of any satisfying experience with his father.

The nurse never saw Mrs. Charles (the mother), but from information given him, including photographs, she was pictured as being large physically, being the dominant person in the home, giving Mr. Charles many contradictory and incompatible messages, and encouraging a symbiotic, dependent relationship between the patient and herself.

One photograph taken during the time of the nurse–patient relationship showed the patient standing between his mother and aunt. In this particular pose, both females were standing very close to the patient, both were taller and broader than the patient, and both had an arm on the patient's closest shoulder extending to the opposite side of his neck. His hands hung at his side, and he stood in a slightly stooped position. The females' smiles were broad and unmistakable; the patient's face gave only the barest trace of a smile.

The following is a letter that Mr. Charles's mother wrote to him and that he voluntarily showed to the nurse.

My poor dear Georgy,

I am working very hard, and I'm tired and miserable. I wish you were home to help me. Why aren't you writing to me? Don't you care about your mother? You're turning out to be just like your father. Is the hospital being good to you? If they aren't, let me know and, by God, they'll hear from me. If you don't write, I won't write to you. You don't care what I'm doing for you. Your father drove me half way to the grave, and you'll probably drive me the rest of the way.

(*signed*)   Your mother

In school Mr. Charles had difficulty learning and was moved from one grade to another largely on social promotions. His main recollections of school were that he was "always made fun of" by his classmates, "especially the boys." He remembered spending much of his time in school "daydreaming." In his sophomore year of high school his illness symptomatology (hallucinations, delusions, persecutory ideas of reference) became acute and caused him to be admitted to a state hospital. The major portion of the remainder of his life up to the age of twenty-one was spent in state hospitals.

At the age of twelve, Mr. Charles, in his own words, "was led into a homosexual act" (fellatio) by a brother-in-law. He claimed that this activity continued for about a year and that he had no further homosexual experiences. However, the hospital records indicated that he had several known homosexual experiences with patients.

In assessing Mr. Charles, the nurse did not consider him to be homosexual in the customary characterological sense. Rather he was considered to be primarily exhibiting problems with self-concept, self-identity, social interactions, and social adjustments of the nature of those of a schizophrenic adaptation. Thus, his past sexual experiences, and especially his concept of himself as "homosexual" were interpreted and treated as part of this schizophrenic process rather than as an unrelated entity.

During the nurse–patient relationship on which this case is based, Mr. Charles demonstrated very little overt evidence of hallucinations, although his history indicated that hallucinations had occurred. They usually centered around religious themes and symbols and had a definite persecutory tone. For example, one auditory and visual hallucination was in the form of a figure of Jesus Christ angrily pointing a finger toward him and shouting, "You are a sinner and will go to hell because you are homosexual." This and similar hallucinations were repeated on various occasions.

Mr. Charles demonstrated some preoccupation with religion and claimed to be very religious, even to the point of considering himself to be a "fanatic." He frequently had the thought that God deliberately made him sick so that he might "do something wonderful for God in the hospital." However, he was not certain what this "wonderful" deed or performance might be. He did think that God might try to visit him in the form of another male patient to give him "instructions." For this reason he "tried to get signs" from newly admitted male patients to see if they might be God.

His only employment had been working as a dishwasher for only a few days at the restaurant where his mother worked as a waitress. He always worked because she wanted him to do so, but only when she would arrange the job for him.

Physical examination revealed no physical pathology or abnormality. The psychiatric diagnosis was "schizophrenic reaction, chronic undifferentiated type."

The nurse in this case was a male and a graduate student in psychiatric nursing. The relationship with Mr. Charles occurred while he was a state hospital inpatient and covered approximately twelve weeks with semiweekly sessions.

Mr. Charles's treatment during this hospitalization included occupational, recreational, and music therapy several times each week. Contact with a psychiatrist was also part of the treatment. However, this physician was the supervisor of the treatment regimen and was not engaged in direct psychotherapy with the patient. Consequently, the physician had only infrequent direct contacts with the patient, and many of those were of a brief, superficial nature. Pharmacologically, various phenothiazine derivatives were incorporated into Mr. Charles's treatment.

The following outline of the nursing care difficulties presented by Mr. Charles and the resultant nursing response is not meant to be inclusive, but rather to give some representative highlights. For convenience, the nurse presents this in the first person.

NURSING PROBLEMS

1. *Difficulty with trust.* In the very first session, after telling me about his "homosexual problem," he asked whether I would tell this to his doctor. I replied that I would if I thought it necessary. The patient's response: "He knows anyway."

Very frequently, especially early in the relationship, he asked me, "You know I trust you, don't you?"

He often asked me if I were "mad" at him. He usually would pick up on some seemingly small aspect in coming to this conclusion, such as when I talked to other patients at times when we did not have an appointment to talk to each other. Also, if I showed the least bit of deviation from our usual interaction pattern (being one minute early or late, walking in a different direction on the sidewalk, having a silence occur).

Problems of trust and dependency also were shown by his numerous questions of, "Do you mind . . . ?" in response to almost everything which we did. ("Do you mind . . . if I talk to you, if we walk here, if I wear this shirt, if I ask this question, if I stop and get a drink, if I look at you, if I cough?")

He interpreted any hesitancy, anxiety, confusion, or frustration on my part as anger toward him, hence, "Are you mad at me?" It should be noted that he was extremely adept in recognizing any of my feelings (real or unreal, although mostly real) that he saw as negative. He consistently referred to himself as the origin and object of these feelings.

In the first few sessions when talking about his "homosexual problem" he was very careful to tell me that he no longer had homosexual "desires." When I missed the clue, he made his point more and more specific until it was inescapable by saying that he never had "desires toward men when I'm in the hospital," that he never had "desires toward staff," and finally that he never had "desires toward anybody in a white uniform." (Now guess who was at this point (1) male, (2) with him in the hospital, (3) part of the "staff," and (4) wearing a white uniform.)

2. *Problems with being overly dependent.* Difficulty trusting and problems with dependency were also evident in his submissive, compliant responses to almost anything which I said in a statement form. Examples include, "Do you mind . . . ?" questions as well as the phrase "Yes, sir." The latter was a response which often followed a statement by me. It usually was not just an affirmative agreement, but seemed to be of a submissive nature, as if he never wanted me to think that he disagreed with me.

NURSING ACTIONS

Tried to be very consistent in all aspects of the relationship. For example, I planned ahead with Mr. Charles the exact date, time, and place of meeting with him. Communication needed to be at concrete levels with utilization of much repetition.

Recognized this as evidence of his concern with trust and his difficulty in trusting me. By implication seemed also to be asking, "Do you trust me?" My response: "It's difficult for two strangers to trust each other. I think you are trying to trust me, and I am trying to trust you."

Asked him what he meant by "mad." Stated factually and concretely, "No, I am not angry at you. If I am angry with you, I will tell you this. Why do you ask? What makes you think that I am angry with you?" (These are examples of responses that were used. These responses were not necessarily used in this sequence or together at the same time.)

Tried to recognize and control my own exasperation at these continuous questions. Gave responses similar to those used in response to his questions of whether I were "mad" at him. "No, I don't mind." "If I don't like . . . or if I don't want to . . . I'll tell you." "Why do you ask?"

Validated this interpretation with the patient. Told him that I did not always know how to respond to him and this sometimes made me feel uncomfortable, but this was not the same as anger toward him. Encouraged the idea of his questioning me. ("This is much better than simply trying to guess what I am thinking or what I mean.")

It is interesting, and perhaps not coincidental, how long it took me to get his message; almost as if I *didn't want* to get his message.

My response: "I think you are telling me that you do have homosexual desires at times toward me. You don't need to be frightened by that because I won't allow any sexual activity to happen between us, and I will still come to see you." His immediate response was to quickly deny that he had any desires toward me; but then he paused, looked up, made eye contact with me and said simply, "Thank you."

This exchange was probably the single most important turning point in his ability to trust me, and equally as important, in my ability to feel comfortable with him.

Began to realize that my responses often promoted his dependent responses, especially when my responses were factual and matter-of-fact, in effect, not encouraging him to make specific choices of his own. Therefore, I began to make a conscious effort to phrase my responses in such a way as to give him the choice of the opinion, or agreement or disagreement when this was appropriate. (From: "I think it's going to rain." To: "It looks as if it might rain. Does it look like that to you?" Or: "Do you think it will rain?")

Concretely protected our relationship by not letting other patients interrupt us when we were talking. This was also helpful in answering his questions about whether I was angry with him and wanted to talk to him.

NURSING PROBLEMS (continued)

Waited for me to make all decisions and apparently expected me to do this.

Wanted to talk only to me.

Patient's response to the idea of termination (subtly expressed hostility toward me, changed various interaction patterns, acute expression of anxiety, attachment to mother and future nursing students).

Continued responses to termination compounded by extreme dependency.

He asked to have a photograph of me (near the end of the relationship).

Patient asked to treat me to a Coke on the last day that we were meeting together. (As we were having our Cokes and hamburgers) patient: "You're giving me more than I'm giving you. The Coke I bought you costs 10 cents and the hamburger you bought me costs 25 cents." (Note concrete thinking.) This was obviously of great importance and concern to the patient.

3. *Problems with inadequate and poorly based self-concept and self-identity.* He thought of himself as "homosexual" and therefore as less than masculine.

"The boys never liked me, they teased me, . . . called me 'queer,' 'sissy,' and 'fairy.' I think they knew that I was a homosexual."

NURSING ACTIONS (continued)

Realized that I was prompting this by making most of the decisions affecting the two of us. Gave him the opportunity as much as I thought was therapeutically helpful to make decisions relating to our relationship.

Examples: Allowed him to decide where I would meet him, where we would go during our sessions, and to some extent what we did (walk, sit, play cards, get Coke, etc.).

Encouraged him to talk to other staff members, students, and patients. Used myself as role model by talking to other patients when we did not have a planned session. As mentioned before, did not allow other patients to interrupt during our planned sessions.

Initiated subject of termination early (in seventh week of twelve-week relationship) in view of his tendency to become very dependent on me. Needed sufficient time to work through feelings evoked when confronted with termination.

Expected these responses through understanding of what termination means to a patient with this illness (total rejection and loss of a global nature). Allowed for expression of feelings, i.e., did not check them, interpret them to patient, or try to change the subject or make light of it. Did not bring up the subject of termination during the next session; gave this opportunity to the patient. (He did bring it up.)

Told the patient that his improvements (enumerated these concretely with him) would be of much greater help to him than my picture. He seemed to accept this and perhaps actually believed it to some extent. If so, note the improvement in abstract, conceptual thinking ability.

Accepted his offer, thanked him, and asked to treat him in return to a hamburger. Nurse: "That's true. I am spending 15 cents more than you are. But you have given me a lot of your time; you have talked to me in spite of sometimes being very uncomfortable, and I think that's worth a lot more than 15 cents. So I don't think at all that I have given you more." In response he smiled, obviously pleased, relieved and satisfied. Again note the concrete to abstract shift.

Reassured him that he was a male. Had him specifically explain what he meant by these various statements and give me examples of when and how the situations occurred.

Helped him to use reality testing to determine just how the boys at school could have known about his limited homosexual activity and that there didn't seem to be any basis in fact for this assumption. ("Did they see you engage in this activity? Did you tell them? Did you engage in this activity with them? Did you actually hear your brother-in-law tell them about your homosexual activities with him?")

NURSING PROBLEMS (continued)

"I wasn't good at sports."
"I was a tattle tale."
"I walk like a girl."

He felt one of the principal reasons he was sick was that he didn't know the "facts of life." His questions left little doubt that he did have very inadequate sexual knowledge, and what he did have was often grossly incorrect. His questions also indicated that he primarily saw male–female interaction at a very primitive, concrete, physical sexual level.

Uncertainty as to how a man thinks, or how he responds in terms of social graces and social expectations.

At first when we approached a door, he waited for me to open it, which I did almost automatically. (Note dependency as well as problems with male social role.)

Waited for me to order Cokes at the canteen (when we had gone there with the purpose of having a Coke).

Apparently did not know when or how to shake hands.

Very unsure of himself in interacting with a female even on a most casual basis.

NURSING ACTIONS *(continued)*

Tried to have him differentiate, by words and walking motion, between the walk of a boy and a girl (he couldn't). "Then how do you know that you walk like a girl?"

Always referred to him as *Mr.* Charles rather than as "Georgy," which he had requested at first. Through this, I hoped to strengthen his identity as a male and adult.

Concretely, factually, and briefly answered his many questions relating to sexual activity, genitalia, and the contribution of these to male–female differences; but in so doing tried to lead him to a more abstract social level of male–female interaction such as friendships, dating, and marriage.

Used myself as a role model to demonstrate male social tasks and male thinking. Also used myself as a "male sounding board."

Encouraged and emphasized his male attributes realistically and included him as a male.

Examples:

Pt.: "It's hard to ask a girl for a date, isn't it?"

Ns.: "Yes, I think so, especially at first. It was hard for me and I think it is hard for most fellows."

Pt.: After going on a pass with his mother to the beach—"I saw some girls in bikinis at the beach. I liked to look at them, do you?"

Ns.: "Yes, I do. I think all guys enjoy that."

Without saying anything to him, I began to hesitate at the doors and he began to open them himself, first with hesitancy, but later with no hesitation.

At first I suggested that he order the Cokes. Later he did this on his own, bringing them over to the table where I was sitting. His reaction indicated that this was a new experience to him, and one which he enjoyed very much.

I always shook hands with him when meeting or leaving him. He began to extend his hand even before I was close enough to shake hands. I also noted that he became very proliferate at shaking hands with other staff members and patients whenever the occasion arose.

One way I attempted to work with this was to prearrange with female classmates for them to join Mr. Charles and myself when we were together but not having a formal session. I would then casually talk with this person, and both of us would try to include Mr. Charles in the conversation. I also had female classmates talk with him at times when I was not there.

On one occasion with my guidance and support, but based on his own initial idea, he invited a female nursing student to his room to share his birthday cake. This was a completely new and unique experience for him as far as dealing socially with a female.

EPILOG

My relationship with Mr. Charles was terminated because of my further educational requirements. At the time of termination, there were no plans for me to have further direct contact with Mr. Charles of any nature, and he was well aware of these conditions.

However, approximately eight weeks after termination, one final contact became unavoidable. I was at this time involved in some practice teaching including clinical supervision of undergraduate nursing students in the psychiatric content area. Out of these responsibilities arose a need for me to make a visit to the hospital where Mr. Charles was a patient. I knew that while a physical meeting with him might be avoidable, my presence at the hospital would most likley be known to him. Therefore, I made arrangements ahead of time to meet with him briefly.

In summary, this meeting seemed rather uncomfortable for both parties. I deliberately tried to keep the interaction on a more superficial level as opposed to the level of intensity during our previous relationship. Mr. Charles appeared as regressed as he had been early in the treatment relationship. He spilled his soft drink, his hands shook, he avoided eye contact, his speech was rapid and halting.

At the end of the visit as we were parting, he did make eye contact and said, "Mr. King, I'm getting worse. I'm backsliding. I'm afraid I'll get sick all over again. I need you to help me." All I could do was remind him of the other staff with whom he had begun to work and his progress which they were reporting.

As I left the hospital, I felt extremely discouraged. It seemed as if all his effort and my effort had been in vain. Psychiatric treatment in general seemed very unproductive, very tenuous, and very unreliable. My sense of accomplishment had evaporated.

However, this setback, if indeed it was one, proved to be only temporary. Through contact with the hospital staff and other nursing students, I learned of Mr. Charles's continuing improvement. He was much more outgoing and spontaneous with people, including females. His level of psychotropic medication was being steadily reduced. His interactions were much more appropriate and apparently rewarding for him. He even came to the point where he could participate in organizing certain patient activities. Finally, my last information was that a trial visit home, including a job, was being planned for and by him.

STUDY GUIDE

Family Relationships

1. Describe the most common personality characteristics of the mother and father of the person experiencing the schizophrenic process.

2. What role do the mother and father play in family functioning as compared to "normal" family role performance?
3. Describe the "climate" of family life.
4. What effect does this type of family relationship have on the child's development of "self-concept?"
5. How does the "double bind communication" contribute to the child's perception of reality—and to all interpersonal relationships?
6. How does the family situation of this child contribute to his development through the dependence-independence struggle?
7. Do all children experiencing the above-mentioned family dynamics develop schizophrenic interpersonal processes?

Pre-psychotic Personality

1. What are some of the characteristics of the schizoid personality?
2. Describe the common interpersonal operations of the schizoid person.
3. What are some of the usual communication patterns seen in persons experiencing the schizophrenic process?
4. What adjustment mechanisms (defense mechanisms) are consistently used?
5. How do social and cultural factors influence this individual?
6. How does the schizoid person cope with the stresses of life?

Nursing Care

1. In Mr. Charles's case, what were the likely roles of his mother and father? What part might these have had in promoting his present illness? What importance does this knowledge have in planning nursing care?
2. What is a delusion? A hallucination? An idea of reference? What might the nurse do if these were presented?
3. How does the nurse promote reality testing and consensual validation?
4. What ability does the schizophrenic patient have to pick up the feelings of others? What type of feeling is the patient most likely to pick up? What implication does this have for nursing care?
5. Is dependency in a patient positive or negative? What might decide this? How does the nurse deal with dependency?
6. What is separation anxiety? Is this normal? How might this be unique with a patient such as Mr. Charles? How might separation anxiety be manifested?
7. What factors might have been involved in the decision of the nurse to to give Mr. Charles a picture of the nurse as was requested? What were possible implications of either giving or not giving the picture?

SELECTED READINGS

C. Aldrich, *An Introduction to Dynamic Psychiatry*, McGraw-Hill, New York, 1966, pp. 250–263.

S. Armstrong, "Thought Disorders of Psychiatric Patients," in Shirley F. Burd and Margaret A. Marshall (eds.), *Some Clinical Approaches to Psychiatric Nursing*, Macmillan, New York, 1963.

J. Haley, "The Art of Being Schizophrenic," *The Power Tactics of Jesus Christ and Other Essays*, Grossman, New York, 1969.

J. Haley, "The Schizophrenic: His Methods and His Therapy," *Strategies of Psychotherapy*, Grune & Stratton, New York, 1963.

G. Laury, "A Schizoid Life Style," *New York State Journal of Medicine*, November 15, 1970, pp. 2809–2814.

T. Lidz *et al.*, *Schizophrenia and the Family*, International Universities Press, New York, 1965.

D. Moser, "Communicating with a Schizophrenic Patient," *Perspectives in Psychiatric Care*, vol. VIII, no. 1, 1970, pp. 36–45.

J. Nehren and N. Gilliam, "Separation Anxiety," *American Journal of Nursing*, vol. 65, January 1965, pp. 109–112.

B. Phillips, "Terminating a Nurse–Patient Relationship," *American Journal of Nursing*, vol. 68, September 1968, pp. 1941–1942.

M. Schwartz and E. Shockley, *The Nurse and the Mental Patient*, Russell Sage Foundation, New York, 1956, pp. 218–281.

S. Smoyak, "Self-Concept and the Schizophrenic Patient," in Shirley F. Burd and Margaret A. Marshall (eds.), *Some Clinical Approaches to Psychiatric Nursing*, Macmillan, New York, 1963.

J. Weakland, "The 'Double-Bind' Hypothesis of Schizophrenia and Three-Party Interaction," in Don D. Jackson (ed.), *The Etiology of Schizophrenia*, Basic Books, New York, 1960.

A. Werner, "Learning to Trust," in Shirley F. Burd and Margaret A. Marshall (eds.), *Some Clinical Approaches to Psychiatric Nursing*, Macmillan, New York, 1963.

Mrs. Kay
twenty-one years old

Ulcerative Colitis/Acute
Lucille D. Gress and Lily Larson

Mrs. Kay is a twenty-one-year-old, frail-looking, tall, thin woman. Her chief complaint on admission was "ulcerative colitis."

Mrs. Kay is the younger of two children. Her brother, twenty-eight years old, has been treated for duodenal ulcers. Her mother, age fifty-five, had a cerebral vascular accident several years ago, but is able to perform her household duties. Mrs. Kay's fifty-eight-year-old father, a bookkeeper, is in fair health (herniated disc; personality change) and reported to be a very passive individual who talks very little. Mrs. Kay described her parents as being very religious, but not overly strict. She said her mother was a very "nervous" person and the "boss" of the family. Mrs. Kay related that generally her home life was pleasant. She expressed annoyance because of her parents' lack of display of affection for each other, and for her and her brother.

Mrs. Kay attended a state college for two years but quit because of problems with "colitis." In January 1971, she was married to a twenty-three-year-old newspaper photographer. Her husband has been treated for duodenal ulcers.

During the admission interview, November 9, 1971, Mrs. Kay said to the nurse, "I appreciate explanations about what's going to happen to me."

The nurse wrote the following on the nursing care Kardex: "A very nervous, apprehensive person. She will need a lot of support and explanation. She has had unpleasant hospital experiences. Since marriage, her colitis has become worse."

PHYSICAL FINDINGS
AND HISTORY (ADMISSION DAY)

Twenty-one-year-old female: chief complaint, chronic ulcerative colitis
Height: 5 feet 8 inches, weight 50 kg (25 kg weight loss since January 1971)
Blood pressure 140/80, pulse 120/minute, respiration 20/minute
Menarche at 12 years, very irregular, 21 to 46 days

Attended college but quit after two years because of colitis
Two years ago she said she had periods of diarrhea and was treated for hook-worm disease by an osteopathic physician. She remained asymptomatic nine months (until May 1971).
July 1971, she returned to the osteopathic hospital with severe diarrhea, temperature 40°C, and anemia. At this point, the diagnosis of ulcerative colitis was made. She was dismissed after several weeks, "in good health," and was told that she was "worrying too much."
September 1971, she developed the "flu" with diarrhea and vomiting. She did not respond to treatment. At this time, red blood appeared in many of her stools.

LABORATORY FINDINGS (ADMISSION DAY)

Urine—routine: pH 4.7, sp. gr. 1.016, glucose negative, protein negative, red blood cells/high power field 1-4, white blood count/high power field 3-5; some mucous threads, some bacteria, occasional hyaline cast.

Blood:
Hemoglobin 6.3 g %
Hematocrit 21
White blood cells/cu mm 14,170
Segmenters 67
Basophils 13
Lymphocytes 9
Monocytes 5
Eosinophils 6
Platelets adequate

Serum—blood group and Rh Factor: A+
Blood urea nitrogen 8 mg %
Sodium 138 meq/liter
Potassium 3.8 meq/liter
Chloride 104 meq/liter
Carbon dioxide (HCO_3) 29 meq/liter
Total proteins 6.4 g %
Albumin 3.0 g %
Globulin 3.0

OTHER LABORATORY VALUES
THROUGHOUT HOSPITALIZATION

Urine

	11/9 Routine	11/11 Routine	12/2 Routine
pH	4.7	5.2	5.0
Specific gravity	1.016	1.014	1.004
Glucose	Negative	Trace—clinistix Negative	Negative
Protein	Negative	Negative	Negative
Red blood cells	1-4		0-2
White blood cells	3-5	2-5	3-4
Microscopic examination	Some mucous threads, some bacteria, occ. hyaline cast, many epithelial cells	Few epithelial cells, moderate bacteria, occasional granular cast	Many calcium oxylate crystals

Blood

	Hgb. g%	Hct. %	W.B.C. cu mm	Seg	Bands	Lym	Mono	Eos	Baso	Platelets
11/9	6.3	21	14,170	67	13	9	5	6		Adequate
11/10	6.8	24.5	10,250	54	17	10	14	4		Adequate
11/11	11.6	36.5	5,890	67	18	8	3			Adequate
11/13	15.8	49.5	11,860	81	7	9	3			Adequate
11/14	16.2	53	14,670	90	3	4	3			Adequate
12/2	13.6	46.5	10,000	76	1	13	7	2	1	Slightly increased
12/7	15.6	44	7,730	65	1	19	10	5		Adequate

Serum—Blood Group and Rh Factor

11/10   A+

	Glucose mg %	Urea N. mg %	Creatinine mg %	Na meq/liter	K meq/liter	Cl meq/liter	CO_2
11/9		8		138	3.8	104	29
11/10	.96	7	1.0				
11/13				142	4.0	103	28
11/16				136	4.6	98	26
11/20				132	4.8	99	23
12/2				141	4.4	97	29
12/7				136	4.3	98	24

MEDICAL ORDERS

11/9   (adm.)
Darvon comp. 65 mg P.O. q. 3 h. p.r.n.
Nembutal 100 mg p.r.n. sleep
Elixir paregoric 10 cc P.O. after loose stool
Lomotil 2.5 mg q. 6 h.
Compazine 10 mg I.M. q. 4 h. p.r.n. nausea
Multivitamins cap. 1 P.O. b.i.d.

11/10
Azulfidine g 1 P.O. q. 6 h.
Decadron 1.5 mg P.O. q. 6 h.
4 units packed cells over next 24 hr

11/11
Valium 5 mg P.O. q. 6 h.
I.V. fluids—1,000 cc of 5% dextrose in distilled water

PREOPERATIVE NURSING— OBJECTIVES AND ACTIONS

11/9, 11/10
The objective of nursing was to assist in controlling diarrhea, decrease nausea and vomiting, assist in increasing hemoglobin and hematocrit values, maintain fluid and electrolyte balance, and provide for appropriate emotional support, a quiet calm environment, and provide physical comfort.

Nausea, vomiting, and diarrhea were gradually diminished by medications. Antibiotics were administered to reduce the bacterial flora of the lower gastrointestinal tract. Mrs. Kay asked for Darvon compound every three hours for joint pain and Nembutal for sleep. Odors from the stool were controlled by careful disposal, deodorant sprays, and thorough cleansing of her bedpan. Mrs. Kay was most meticulous about her own cleanliness and used colognes and bath powder frequently after washing.

The nurse explained to Mrs. Kay the reasons for the medical regime and reinforced the explanations of colectomy and ileostomy. Mrs. Kay was a most interested listener, and at that time, talked about her physiologic functions in a very detached way, as though her body were not a part of herself and that the surgery was really not going to happen to her. The nurse who admitted Mrs. Kay became Mrs. Kay's nurse for the day shift during the entire preoperative period. The nurse decided that Mrs. Kay needed someone she could relate to and someone to help her gradually overcome her "denial" of reality. Mrs. Kay revealed to the

nurse that she thought her marriage was in jeopardy because of her illness and that her husband really did not overtly show much affection for
her. "He doesn't kiss me very often nor even tell me he loves me." The
nurse listened carefully and helped Mrs. Kay examine her own feelings.
Mrs. Kay, on the second hospital day, said in an angry, hurt manner,
"My husband just doesn't care. He hasn't been to see me yet." The nurse
asked if he were working and suggested that the long travel distance
might have prevented him from visiting her. The nurse asked Mrs. Kay
if she had spoken to him on the telephone and suggested that he might
be quite worried about her. Just before the nurse was to go off duty, she
stopped to see Mrs. Kay, whose husband had arrived. Mrs. Kay asked
the nurse if she would help her explain "all about an ileostomy to my
husband." Mr. Kay appeared very shy but the nurse asked what the
physician had explained to him. He said, "All I know is that Millie's
going to have all her bowel removed and that she won't be able to control
her stool."

The nurse showed some simple anatomical illustrations of an ileostomy stoma and explained how persons learn to adjust and carry on
activities after the surgical scar is healed. The nurse explained about the
local ileostomy-colostomy club and offered to call a member, a young
married woman who had an ileostomy two years ago and who visited
patients. Both Mr. and Mrs. Kay approved of the "ileostomy" visitor
coming before surgery. The nurse also explained reasons for the medicines Mrs. Kay was receiving preoperatively.

11/11
Mrs. Kay has an intellectual understanding of her medical problem and
understands the reasons for an ileostomy and feels that an ileostomy is
better "than living the way I have the past year." Diarrhea was controlled
to three stools over the past twenty-four hours. There was less bleeding,
but the stool was still tinged with blood.

11/12
Physician's progress notes: Physical condition indicates ready for surgery.
Hemoglobin and hematocrit too low for surgery. Will give 1 unit of packed
cells today.

11/12
Physician's orders:
  1 unit packed cells today
  Pre-op med. on call for 11/13:
    Demerol 50 mg
    Phenergan 25 mg   I.M.
    Atropine 0.4 mg

11/12
Nurse's observations and activities. Mrs. Kay appeared more anxious the day before surgery. The nurse decided that she would sit quietly with Mrs. Kay, as she expressed hostility toward both nurses and physicians. Mrs. Kay verbalized her fears of becoming an invalid, fears that her husband would find her unattractive, and how they could not meet hospitalization and physician costs. The nurse and Mrs. Kay set the first priorities to be "avoidance of becoming an invalid," and that the other problem could be faced more productively if she, together with her husband, and the medical and nursing staff, would focus on alleviating her health problem. The nurse decided that this was an opportune time to have Mrs. Kay practice deep breathing, coughing, turning in bed, and she explained the importance of Mrs. Kay's participation. She explained to Mrs. Kay where the incisions would be (abdominal and pereneal) and showed Mrs. Kay an ileostomy bag, its function, and where it would be placed. She also explained that Mrs. Kay would have I.V.s and a Foley catheter and a nasogastric tube, which would be placed before surgery. The nurse felt that Mrs. Kay had a good understanding of the reasons for this preparation and knew that nurses and doctors would be present to care for her. Mrs. Kay expressed concern about the lack of attention during the evening and night and that her light was not answered for "hours." The nurse placed on the Kardex, "Mrs. Kay is a very frightened woman. Give backrub at bedtime, check her frequently. Most of all she needs to know we care."

OPERATION (FOURTH DAY AFTER ADMISSION)

Total colectomy, permanent ileostomy, proctectomy, penrose drain in rectal wound sutured to skin. Perineal dressings with "T" binder applied.

FINAL DIAGNOSIS

The final diagnosis was granulomatous ulcerative colitis.

11/13
Post-op: Foley to D.D.
I&O—including ileostomy drainage
N.P.O.—I.V. fluids—1,000 cc of 5% dextrose in distilled water—
with 40 meq KCl
Cough/D.B. q. 2 h.
Ampicillin 500 mg q. 6 h. via volutrol

11/13
Streptomycin 500 mg I.M. q. 12 h. x6 days
Decadron 4 mg I.M. q. 6 h.

C.B.C. and electrolytes
1 unit whole blood
Irrigate N.G. tube
Change perineal dressing

11/14
D.C. Foley
I.V. fluids

11/15
Culture and sensitivity (C&S)—urine
Clear liquids and I.V. fluids until further notice

11/13–15
Nursing observations and actions. Careful monitoring of intravenous fluids as ordered. Accurate monitoring and recording of urinary and ileal stoma output, and gastric content through the nasogastric tube. Irrigation of nasogastric tube with normal saline as needed for patency. Protection of the skin around ileal stoma by cleaning, drying, and applying tincture of benzoin to the dry skin directly around the stoma before applying temporary bag. The stoma bag opening was carefully measured and cut so the adhesive portion covered the entire skin around the stoma.

Copious amount of fluid from the stoma was collected in a urine bag, which was attached by means of sterile tubing placed in the lower end of the ostomy bag. This kept the weight of the ostomy bag from pulling the adhesive off the surrounding skin, thus preventing the contents of the ileum from spilling on the skin.

11/14
Nursing observation and actions. The nasogastric tube was removed. Mrs. Kay was encouraged to take clear liquids, which she tolerated. Pereneal dressings were changed; there was a moderate amount of serosanguineous drainage.

11/15
Full liquid diet was not tolerated. Mrs. Kay became nauseated and vomited at every attempt to take even clear liquids. Temperature increased from 38.4°C. to 39°C. Intravenous fluids were increased to 3,000 cc for the next twenty-four hours. Mrs. Kay frequently examined her ileostomy bag and said, "Can you imagine carrying this around all my life!" Perineal dressings were changed.

11/16
Urine output per voiding 150 cc or less. Mrs. Kay complained of burning of perineium during and following voiding.

11/16
Physician's orders:
  N.P.O.
  Normal saline I.V. with 40 meq KCl x2
  Reinsert Foley catheter

11/16
Nursing observations and actions. Foley catheter to direct closed drainage. 500 cc residual urine obtained. Temperature 38.4°C. Mrs. Kay says she has the "flu," had one shaking chill after which temperature reached 39.4°C. Mrs. Kay continues to require Compazine for nausea and vomiting.

11/16
Nursing observations. Perineal dressings have a small amount of serous drainage. Laparotomy incision is clean, exposed to air. Skin about the stoma remains intact—no excoriation. Mrs. Kay walked about in her room, emptied and measured drainage from the ostomy bag. She put on makeup today after assistance with bathing. She tolerates liquids only in small amounts. Mrs. Kay requires medications for nausea and vomiting after removal of the nasogastric tube. She has many requests of the staff, especially during the evening and night. Some of the staff felt she was an unreasonable and demanding patient. Mrs. Kay informed her day nurse that one nurse at night told her that she acted like a baby.

11/17
Nursing and medical conference. The nurse caring for Mrs. Kay during the day met with the evening staff and the physician to discuss Mrs. Kay's nursing needs and how the staff might approach Mrs. Kay in the best possible way.

One nurse said, "She's a very intelligent young woman with much feeling for people. She knows that she has annoyed some of the nurses, but says she can't help it. We should be very careful not to upset her. It seems she gets more nauseated when she has to wait for her light to be answered."

The physician stated that her physical condition may contribute to her impatience. Her radical surgical procedure has also been a shock. Nurses discussed their feelings about Mrs. Kay and decided that a more positive approach could be taken by all staff.

11/19
The nursing staff who worked with Mrs. Kay found that their visits and attentions with her were rewarding both to Mrs. Kay and to the staff. She felt that the staff understood her requests and as a result she said she was more tolerable to them.

Mrs. Kay needed assistance for several days in ambulating, as her muscle strength had diminished since her hospitalization. Her weight was 50.5 kg, 0.5 kg above her admission weight.

PHYSICIAN'S ORDERS

11/18
I.V. with 40 meq. KCl x2

11/19
I.V. fluids with 20 meq. KCl
D.C. Ampicillin and strep.
D.C. I.V.

11/21
Release clamp on Foley q. 4 h. for 30 min and reclamp
Sitz baths

11/24
Hi-pro, lo-residue diet
Decadron 0.5 mg P.O. b.i.d.
Valium 2.5 mg P.O. t.i.d.

11/25
D.C. Foley—Urine culture and sensitivity
Myocholine 25 mg P.O.—1st dose, then 10 mg P.O. q. 6 h.
Residual urine 500 cc

11/26
Reinsert Foley catheter—do not clamp—open at all times
Furadantin 100 mg P.O. q. 6 h.

11/30
Neosynephrine nose gtts. ii q.i.d. x3 days
Sucret lozenges
Vaporizer

12/1
C.B.C.—electrolytes
Compazine 10 mg P.O. q. 6 h. nausea

12/3
D.C. Foley (U.A.)
Myocholine 50 mg P.O. q. 6 h.
May take shower

LATER POSTOPERATIVE PERIOD PROGRESS

Mrs. Kay had some urinary tract infection, the "flu," and separation of the perineal wound. She was placed on a selective regular diet to enable her to choose foods she liked. Her appetite fluctuated, but she took the initiative to drink fluids of all kinds to help counteract the urinary tract infection. When the Foley catheter was removed, Mrs. Kay had a residual urine of 500 cc due to an atonic bladder. A Foley catheter was reinserted and mediation given for the infection. The "flu" was treated symptomatically. During this episode, her ileostomy was very active. She became quite adept at caring for her ostomy appliance, but was dissatisfied with it and requested to see the Ostomy Appliance representative. She chose a bag that would be better concealed under her clothing.

11/21–26
Nursing objectives and actions. Continue assisting Mrs. Kay to care for her ileostomy and explain why she has more liquid from the ileostomy. Sometimes to assist with Sitz bath, and observe her dilate stoma daily. Provide for rest. Encourage fluids to 3,000 cc per day. Offer high protein snacks between meals. Likes milk shakes with an egg, beef broth, and cranberry juice. Give medication for urinary infection. Encourage her to order high protein foods. Perineal wound granulating and clean—minimal drainage. Reinsert Foley catheter (residual urine 300 cc). Temperature between 37.5–38°C.

11/27–28
Nursing observations. Diminished fluid output from ileostomy. Intake adequate, output adequate. Mrs. Kay is in good spirits, walks in the hall, and visits with patients carrying her urine bag.

11/29
Nursing observations and actions. Mrs. Kay feels chilly and feverish, has a sore throat.

11/30
Medications and vaporizer used for upper respiratory infection. Mrs. Kay is concerned about "all my infections." Nursing staff asked Mrs. Kay not to visit patients for a while until her upper respiratory infection is cleared.

12/1
Mrs. Kay again is nauseated, relieved with Compazine.

12/3
Nursing observations, goals, and actions. Mrs. Kay said, "I feel better than I have for years." Her weight gain since admission was 2 kg, her physical condition stable. There was 50 cc of residual urine after the Foley catheter was removed. Temperature is normal.

To help Mrs. Kay with diet intake, choose foods which are high protein, high caloric, and low residue.

Mrs. Kay is concerned about her future relationship with her husband.

12/5
Mrs. Kay requested a psychiatric consultation. She felt that this consultation would help both her and her husband.

Psychiatric consultation (approximately one month after admission and the day before discharge from the hospital). The psychiatrist added the following note to the chart.

Addendum to medical history. "Last two years had ulcerative colitis." It has been worse at times when she was under pressure (work, study, etc.). Gives history of depression during her senior year in high school due to people not accepting her change from an introverted to an extroverted kind of person. At this time, she took an overdose of tranquilizers. Doubts herself that she wanted to die. Since then she has been depressed only when feeling ill, but never had suicidal thoughts, except once when she had a big quarrel with her husband. "Says she has 'hangups,' one which is being oversensitive about the suffering of children in Biafra and Vietnam, the other one refers to her husband being undemonstrative and not showing affection. (They have been married almost a year and have had sex relations perhaps twenty times.) She gives the impression of continual role-playing."

Impression. Hysterical personality.

Recommend. (1) individual or group psychotherapy; (2) marriage counseling. Both of the above could be obtained in her home town.

During the last week of Mrs. Kay's hospital stay, the nursing staff were regular visitors in her room. On morning rounds, Mrs. Kay had some new incident to relate or some new drawing or clipping to show the staff. She walked the halls frequently with her urine bag in one hand, and waving with the other. No one seemed too busy to talk with her.

Upon discharge, Mrs. Kay presented a large humorous poster apologizing for her being "a trying patient." She thanked the medical and nursing staff for their patience. The attractive picture poster remained on the bulletin board on the unit for several weeks.

PROGRESS NOTES FOLLOWING HOSPITAL DISMISSAL

12/9
Dismissed

Return to clinic in one month
Myocholine 50 mg q. 6 h.

Furadantin 100 mg q. 6 h.
Valium 2.5 mg p.r.n.
Dramamine 50 mg p.r.n.

1/9/72
Weight gain 2.7 kg over admission weight.

JUNE 1972

The head nurse received a letter from Mrs. Kay. The following excerpts are taken from the letter:

"I am sorry to have neglected my favorite people at the university hospital.

"I think I can go back as a nurse's aide where I worked before but don't think I'm ready to lift yet. So far the last few months I've been at a sewing factory running a sewing machine. It pays well, which I need for all the medical bills to pay.

"I just finished designing and decorating a three-tier wedding cake for one of my friends and my dear husband helped put it together. I think we should begin a business of our own.

"We had to move into another apartment because the other building had to be razed. They have sold this one so will have to look again. We have another dog—he adopted us so our house in every room has dog hairs, bones, and dirty dog tracks. We still love him.

"I talked with a nursing instructor, and she wants me to talk to students so they can understand what an 'ostomy' is all about.

"If I can help you in any way, I'm still available, and on call.

"Please give my regards to your very nice nursing staff and give a great big hug to Dr. Howe and Dr. Thomas from me."

STUDY GUIDE

1. What was the relationship, if any, between Mrs. Kay's family, social and personal life, and her medical problem(s)?
2. What individuals are most susceptible to ulcerative colitis? How did Mrs. Kay's situation compare with findings reported in the literature?
3. What are the developmental tasks normally ascribed to the individual in Mrs. Kay's developmental stage? How were her health problem(s) likely to affect achievement of these tasks?

4. What were the pertinent objectives of the preoperative nursing care in this case?
5. Identify the significant data in this case and relate the findings to the specific objectives of the preoperative plan of care (anxiety level, laboratory reports, etc.).
6. What were appropriate objectives for the postoperative care on the case? (Review the report of the first, second, third and fourth postoperative days.)
7. What may be contributory factors related to the complications (wound infection, urinary tract infection, urinary retention) in the immediate postoperative period and later during her upper respiratory infection?
8. Explain the rationale for the medical, pharmacological, and dietary regimen prescribed for Mrs. Kay.
9. What was Mrs. Kay's response to treatment? How does her response compare to an "uncomplicated" case?
10. What should be incorporated into the plan of nursing action related to continuity of care (caring for the "ostomy," source of supplies, activities, etc.)?
11. Compare the care of the person with an ileostomy with that of the individual with a colostomy. How does the loss of electrolytes from the upper gastrointestinal tract differ in its effect on the patient from those lost from the lower gastrointestinal tract?

SELECTED READINGS

I. L. Beland, *Clinical Nursing*, Macmillan, New York, 1965, pp. 105–106, 525–526.

L. S. Brunner *et al.*, *Textbook of Medical-Surgical Nursing*, 2nd ed. J. B. Lippincott, Philadelphia, 1970, pp. 483–486.

Colostomy, Ileostomy and Ureterostomy: A Guide of Practical Information for Nurses, rev. ed. American Cancer Society, Inc., Cuyahoga Unit, Ohio Division, 1970.

G. E. Gibbs and Marilyn White, "Stomal Care," *American Journal of Nursing*, vol. 72, no. 2, February 1972, pp. 268–271.

F. Gutowski, "Ostomy Procedure: Nursing Care Before and After," *American Journal of Nursing*, vol. 72, no. 2, February 1972, pp. 262–267.

E. A. Katona, "Learning Colostomy Control," *American Journal of Nursing*, March 1967, pp. 534–541.

N. M. Metheney and W. D. Snively, *Nurses Handbook of Fluid Balance*, J. B. Lippincott, Philadelphia, 1967.

H. S. Mitchell *et al.*, *Cooper's Nutrition in Health and Disease*, 15th ed. J. B. Lippincott, Philadelphia, 1968, pp. 382–384.

Mrs. Pratt
twenty-three years old

Threatened Abortion/Acute
Betty L. Wilkerson and Rosemary Cannon Kilker

ADMISSION

It was late afternoon when Mrs. Pratt, twenty-three years old, Gravida i, was admitted into the emergency room. She was crying uncontrollably and her husband seemed unable to comfort her. The patient had been referred to the hospital by her private physician with the diagnosis of threatened abortion. Her last menstrual period had been eight weeks previously.

As the nurse was removing Mrs. Pratt's blood-soaked garments, two sanitary pads, and a turkish towel, Mrs. Pratt continually asked, "Will the bleeding stop?" "Will I lose the baby?" The nurse replied, "I know you are afraid. The bleeding will be stopped, but it is likely you will lose the baby."

Vital signs were taken by the nurse and intravenous fluids were started. The patient was positioned for a pelvic exam. After the physician removed clots from the vagina, he found the cervix dilated 2 cm with membranes glistening. The nurse remained at the patient's side with her hand resting on Mrs. Pratt's shoulder during the examination. Arrangements were made for an emergency dilatation and curettage. An explanation was quickly given to Mr. and Mrs. Pratt by the physician. Following the dilatation and curettage, the patient was transferred to a two-bed room on a gynecological unit. Routine postoperative observations were carried out.

While caring for Mrs. Pratt, the nurse learned how much she had desired this baby. Mrs. Pratt told of how she and her husband had decided to discontinue the use of contraceptives six months previously and how excited they were to have the pregnancy confirmed. Mrs. Pratt was still teaching kindergarten, as her physician had told her that her health and the pregnancy appeared normal and that she should continue her usual activities. Mrs. Pratt was happy about this, as she enjoyed teaching and the curiosity of young children. She is now wondering if whether she had quit work this would have made a difference in being able to carry the baby. The nurse reaffirmed what the physician had told the Pratts—that he had found no evidence of infection or disease of the endometrium, no cervical incompetence, or other physical reasons for the miscarriage. The nurse also told the couple that it is a normal reaction for a woman to blame herself, but that Mrs. Pratt must realize that the miscarriage occurred for unexplained reasons.

During visiting hours, the Pratts asked the nurse to answer some questions they had forgotten to ask the physician. How soon could Mrs. Pratt resume teaching, and how soon could she attempt another pregnancy? The nurse said the physician would be seeing her in the morning before she was dismissed and would give her his dismissal recommendations, but she believed he would advise her to stay at home about a week, to rest and take it easy, and, then, by all means to continue teaching. The nurse also said that it should be about six months before they should attempt another pregnancy. Mrs. Pratt asked if she should start taking the "pill" again, and the nurse answered that she felt it would be best for the physician to advise her concerning resumption of the birth control pill. The nurse mentioned that sexual intercourse could usually be resumed after ten to fourteen days. Mrs. Pratt had an uneventful recovery and was dismissed in twenty-four hours.

PHYSICIAN'S ORDERS ON ADMISSION

1. C.B.C.
2. Type and cross match, set up 2 units blood
3. Fibrinogen level
4. Start 5% Ringers lactate I.V.
5. Pre-op for emergency D&C

POST-OP ORDERS

1. Vital signs every 15 min until stable
2. Check for bleeding
3. Demerol 50 mg I.M. p.r.n. for pain
4. Catheterize if unable to void in 8 hr
5. Ambulate in 4 hr
6. Seconal 100 mg P.O.—H.S.
7. Regular diet
8. Hemoglobin, hematocrit in A.M.
9. D.C. present I.V. when infused

STUDY GUIDE

1. Why would a nurse respond to a patient, "I know you are afraid?"
2. How would you classify Mrs. Pratt's abortion?

3. Why is a D&C necessary in Mrs. Pratt's case?
4. What safety factors must be utilized in the nursing care of Mrs. Pratt returning to the unit directly from surgery?
5. What physiological readjustments occur following an abortion?
6. Discuss the social information given as it relates to the psychological readjustments following an abortion.
7. How can the nurse support and reassure Mr. and Mrs. Pratt during the abortion?
8. What are some of the common causes of spontaneous abortion?
9. How can the nurse best answer the patient's question, "Will I abort again?"

SELECTED READINGS

E. Fitzpatrick *et al.*, *Maternity Nursing*, J. B. Lippincott, Philadelphia and Toronto, 1971, pp. 458–462.

F. Goodrich, "Obstetric Hemorrhage," *American Journal of Nursing*, November 1962, pp. 96–97.

L. M. Hellman and J. Pritchard, *Williams Obstetrics*, 14th ed., Appleton-Century-Crofts, New York, 1971, pp. 504–519.

S. Olds, "What We Do—and Don't Know About Miscarriage," *Today's Health*, February 1971, pp. 42–45.

J. Tucker, "Nursing Care in Obstetric Hemorrhage," *American Journal of Nursing*, November 1962, pp. 98–101.

Mrs. Sparks
twenty-eight years old

Placenta Previa/Acute
Rosemary Cannon Kilker and Betty L. Wilkerson

ADMISSION

An extremely pale young woman was wheeled by cart into the admissions room of the labor and delivery department. She was accompanied by her husband who stammered to the nurse, "She's bleeding again—only this time a lot of it."

NURSE'S ACTIONS

The nurse quickly introduced herself to the couple and assisted Mrs. Sparks to the examining table. She directed Mr. Sparks to the waiting room until his wife was admitted. While she was assisting Mrs. Sparks in undressing and gowning, she ascertained the following information: twenty-eight years old, Gravida v, Para iv, thirty-six weeks gestation, last pregnancy eighteen months ago, past obstetrical history noncontributory except for one week previous when she had a brief period of painless spotting.

Mrs. Sparks's blood pressure was 90/50, pulse 120. She complained of thirst and was apprehensive. Mrs. Sparks estimated she had lost three cups of bright blood at home and at present had a bath towel well saturated. The nurse alerted the house physician to come at once. Further assessment revealed a soft uterus, fetal heart rate 140/minute, and the fetus lying in the transverse position. No uterine contractions were felt, and the patient stated she had felt no discomfort or pain.

PHYSICIAN'S ORDERS

The physician concurred with the nurse's findings and ordered a stat hemoglobin, which revealed 10 g, hematocrit value of 29%, and urinalysis negative for sugar and protein.

Further orders were: nothing by mouth, bed rest, Foley catheter to dependent drainage, type and cross match for four units of blood, prepare for double set up (cesarean and vaginal delivery), fibrinogen count, 1,000 cc 5% Ringers Lactate I.V.

The physician then explained the diagnosis, possible placenta previa, to Mr. and Mrs. Sparks and suggested that Mr. Sparks wait in the waiting room until he or the nurse could notify him further of his wife's situation.

MEDICAL TREATMENT

Twenty minutes after admission, Mrs. Sparks was taken to the operative delivery room where she was prepared for surgery. A sterile vaginal examination was done. It revealed the cervix to be 2 cm dilated, uneffaced, and sponge-like tissue was felt covering the internal os. A small amount of bright red bleeding resulted from the examination. Under general anesthetic, a cesarean was performed. A live-born baby girl was delivered with an Apgar of 6 at 1 minute, and 9 at 5 minutes. Her birth weight was 2.33 kg. The placenta was found to be completely obstructing the cervical os. Three units of blood were given stat postoperatively.

NURSE'S ACTIONS

The nurse sent word to Mr. Sparks while the cesarean was occurring, and he was shown his new daughter while she was en route to the premature nursery. Immediate postoperative care proved uneventful.

Nursing care of the first postoperative postpartum day combined physical and emotional support. To meet the mother's needs to receive an abundance of emotional replenishment and physical relaxation, the nursing interaction consisted of a complete bed bath and perineal care. While doing the eight-point postpartal check,* the nurse chatted with Mrs. Sparks concerning her self-care and body changes. Following the check, the nurse felt that Mrs. Sparks needed the opportunity to discuss the crisis situation and emergency surgery. The nurse was best able to do this by sitting with the patient.

Later postpartal care included premature and general infant care, sibling rivalry, and family planning. Special attention was given to encourage the "mothering" process, since the infant might be staying a few days after Mrs. Sparks's dismissal. Arrangements were completed for follow-up nursing care in the home.

STUDY GUIDE

1. Discuss the etiology of placenta previa.
2. What are the signs of placenta previa?

---

* See eight-point check in this book in the case of Miss Blackwell, pp. 75–76

3. What is and is not included in the nursing assessment of Mrs. Sparks?
4. What are the anticipated nursing actions in the initial care of Mrs. Sparks?
5. Is there much fluctuation in the fibrinogen count at this time? Why or why not?
6. Assess the following nursing situation. 2:00 A.M.: You are the nurse in charge of a labor area. A Gravida ii, Para i mother, thirty-six weeks gestation, in active labor, begins to have a greater amount of bloody show than you consider normal. She has no acute pain or discomfort. Fetal heart rate is normal, vital signs are normal. Her private physician is not in the hospital. What would be your nursing actions?
7. What emergency equipment would you have in readiness for the above situation? How would you best answer the mother's question "Is my baby going to die? Will I be all right?"
8. What anticipatory planning is necessary for the care of this newborn?

SELECTED READINGS

J. Beazley, "Inevitable Antepartum Hemorrhage," *Nursing Times*, August 12, 1971, pp. 985–987.

W. H. Blahd, *Nuclear Medicine*, 2nd ed., McGraw-Hill, New York, 1971, pp. 517–519.

B. Drukker *et al.*, "Placental Localization," *American Journal of OB and GYN*, May 1, 1971, pp. 9–13.

E. Fitzpatrick, *et al.*, *Maternity Nursing*, J. B. Lippincott, Philadelphia and Toronto, 1971, pp. 466–468, 485–489, 495–500, 505–506.

F. Goodrich, "Obstetric Hemorrhage," *American Journal of Nursing*, November 1962, pp. 96–97.

L. M. Hellman and J. Pritchard, *Williams Obstetrics*, 14th ed., Appleton-Century-Crofts, New York, 1971, pp. 609–635.

E. H. Hon, *An Introduction to Fetal Heart Rate Monitoring*, Harty Press, New Haven, Conn., 1971.

C. Lasater, "Electronic Monitoring of Mother and Fetus," *American Journal of Nursing*, April 1972, pp. 728–730.

J. Tucker, "Nursing Care in Obstetric Hemorrhage," *American Journal of Nursing*, November 1962, pp. 98–101.

J. Turbeville, "Nurse's Role in Hospital Care," *Hospital Topics*, June 1972, pp. 85–88, 103.

Mr. Alden
thirty-four years old

Alcoholism|Acute and Chronic
Sandra Tweed Blades

INTRODUCTION

Mr. Tim Alden is thirty-four years old. He grew up in a small town in southern Kansas where he now works as a postal clerk. He has been married to Carol for twelve years. They have six children. Three of the children are from two previous marriages of Carol's, and Tim has legally adopted them. The children range in age from six to seventeen years. From a distance, they would appear to be a normal family with the usual day-to-day problems of life. However, some of their closer friends and their minister realize that this is not the case, because Tim is an alcoholic.

Mr. Alden had his first drink when he was eighteen years old. He remembers well the good feeling he got from that drink. He continued to drink occasionally "with the guys." A couple of years later he went into the Navy. He was in the Navy four years and drank quite heavily. His drinking decreased more to "normal" when he returned home after discharge. However, it has become an increasing problem the last eight years, and during the last three years Mr. Alden has gone only one to two days without drinking several beers and some whiskey.

Mr. Alden was admitted to an alcoholism treatment center on September 8 at 3 A.M. He was brought in by his minister and a member of Alcoholics Anonymous. During the previous day, Mr. Alden had worked as usual at the post office. On his way home he had stopped for several drinks and had purchased a bottle of whiskey. When he got home at about 7 P.M., Mrs. Alden let him know that she was angry at his being late. About an hour later, Mrs. Alden went to her job as a waitress. Shortly thereafter, Mr. Alden called her to come home because he knew there was something wrong and he needed help. When she arrived, Mr. Alden had secluded himself upstairs in the house. He would allow no one to go up, throwing furniture down at anyone who tried going up to see him. Mrs. Alden called several Alcoholics Anonymous members, their minister, and their doctor. Finally, Mr. Alden was calmed down and brought sixty miles to the alcoholism treatment center. Mr. Alden had had his last drink about one and one-half hours before admission. He was rational and was placed in the emergency bed for observation.

NURSING HISTORY (TAKEN FROM MR. AND MRS. ALDEN ON SEPTEMBER 12)

Presenting Problem

"Can't handle my drinking."

History of Present and Past Health

Ruptured appendix—five years old
Asthma in childhood
Bleeding ulcers ten years ago; treated at Veterans Administration hospital
No drug allergies
No history of convulsions of DTs

The patient stated he had had a problem with alcohol for sixteen years. He was treated three years ago at a "mental clinic" in a large city for three weeks, where he was told by a psychiatrist that he was an alcoholic. While in treatment, he was allowed off the ward three times, and each time he continued to drink.

Regarding the night of admission, the patient stated that he does not remember what happened after calling his wife to come home from work.

Mr. Alden stated that he had been involved in Alcoholics Anonymous for a short period of time several years ago.

Family History

Father.
deceased of heart attack two years ago

Mother.
sixty-two years old, heart trouble

Five brothers.
two have drinking problems

One sister.
Mr. Alden's mother comes to him often for advice and he makes recommendations to her, which often upset his brothers and sister. Also, she is con-

sidering moving a trailer home to a lot across the street from the Alden's "if Carol doesn't want me moving in with you."

Social History

Tim and Carol's social activity has deteriorated because he prefers to go where liquor is being served and she is no longer inclined to participate in his drinking activities. They have no mutual close friends. They both seem to realize that they have channeled their social relationships in different directions.

Tim used to be a Boy Scout leader and quite active in the Methodist Church. However, his activities in both these organizations have dwindled. Sporadically, he and Carol do continue to attend a couples group from the Church that meets weekly. As a family group they do not do as many things together as they used to.

PSYCHOLOGICAL TESTING (REPORT OF THE PSYCHOLOGIST)

Shipley Hartford

Mr. Alden's I.Q. is 117 (upper limits of bright average category). His abstract ability is excellent. Mr. Alden should have no difficulty in reasoning or understanding the treatment program.

Bender Gestalt Test

Adequately done. There are some indications of collision tendencies, suggestive of the possibility of emotional disturbances. The test was also quite well organized and tends to indicate some very strong perfectionist tendencies.

Rotter Incomplete Sentence Test

This test substantiates the perfectionism. There is a great deal of worry and concern about his drinking and he appears to be quite well motivated to stop his drinking. He admits that his nerves are very poor and that he wants to be better. He has a poor self-concept. He appears to be rather withdrawn and filled with psychological tensions. He is particularly worried about his financial affairs. This man is trying desperately not to run from himself, and yet tension is building to such a point that it is possible he will run.

MMPI

This test shows an individual who has almost every psychiatric symptom that can show up on the test. He is a very sick man. He appears to be severely neurotic, but some psychotic personality patterns show up. Perfectionism is extremely high. He needs to do everything just perfectly. This test also shows a flight of ideas. Mr. Alden's thinking is extremely confused and could border on being bizarre. He is also a very sensitive individual. He is impulsive and tends to react on the spur of the moment and has difficulty learning from past experience. Depression is also evident in the overall personality pattern. He is trying to handle some of his difficulties with the utilization of projection. He also uses physical complaints as a method of reducing his tension. To make this matter more difficult, he is an introverted person who keeps all his problems bottled up inside himself, and it will be very difficult for him to establish a trusting relationship.

Diagnostic Impression
Alcoholism

Prognosis
Guarded

CHAPLAIN'S REPORT
Mr. Alden's religious background is Methodist. In high school he had thoughts of entering the ministry. He said that he has had difficulty with Step 3 of the Alcoholics Anonymous program, because he has not been able to think of God as a loving God. It seems that he is "projecting" a great deal—blaming others (including God) for his troubles.

PHYSICAL EXAMINATION AND LABORATORY TESTS

Height: 5 ft., 8 in.; *weight:* 67.3 kg

B.P.: 120/80; *pulse:* 72

Abdomen: Soft—liver not enlarged

Chest x ray: Normal

V.D.R.L.: Nonreactive

Hemoglobin: 17.6 g%

Hematocrit: 53%

W.C./cmm: 6,000

Glucose: 92 mg%

BUN: 24 mg%

Alkaline phosphate: 1.0

Cholesterol: 304 mg%

Thymol turbidity: 2.2

Total protein: 8.8 g%

Albumin: 4.5 g%

Globulin: 4.3 g%

A/G ratio: 1.0

Uric acid: 3.7

THE TWELVE STEPS OF ALCOHOLICS ANONYMOUS

1. We admitted we were powerless over alcohol—that our lives had become unmanageable.
2. Came to believe that a Power greater than ourselves could restore us to sanity.
3. Made a decision to turn our will and our lives over to the care of God *as we understood Him.*
4. Made a searching and fearless moral inventory of ourselves.
5. Admitted to God, to ourselves, and to another human being the exact nature of our wrongs.
6. Were entirely ready to have God remove all these defects of character.
7. Humbly asked Him to remove our shortcomings.
8. Made a list of all persons we had harmed, and became willing to make amends to them all.
9. Made direct amends to such people wherever possible, except when to do so would injure them or others.
10. Continued to take personal inventory and when we were wrong promptly admitted it.
11. Sought through prayer and meditation to improve our conscious contact with God *as we understood Him*, praying only for knowledge of His will for us and the power to carry that out.
12. Having had a spiritual awakening as the result of these steps, we tried to carry this message to alcoholics, and to practice these principles in all our affairs.

HOSPITAL COURSE

9/8   3 A.M.

Patient admitted in rational state to emergency bed.

Patient asked if he had medication or alcoholic beverages with him. Stated "no."

Observed for delirium tremens (DTs). Librium was given intramuscularly and a quiet environment was provided for the patient to rest. The patient did not develop hallucinosis or DTs. Observations that would have indicated these problems are severe apprehension, restlessness, and misrepresentation of the environment. DTs usually develop within the first 48 hours after withdrawal from alcohol.

5 A.M.
Patient vomiting—has not slept yet.

6–12 P.M.
Sleeping.

12–8 P.M.
Visiting with other patients. Patient appears shaky. Librium was given orally. (Librium was given four times a day for a week to help calm the patient and to prevent DTs.)

8 P.M.
Patient went to bed stating he thought he could sleep without sleeping medication.

9/9
Physical exam and lab tests. Physical problems common to alcoholics include cirrhosis of the liver, esophageal varicies, gastritis, pancreatitis, and nutritional deficiencies. Mr. Alden's physical examination and lab tests did not show that any of these problems were present.

Psychological testing was administered.

9/10
Therapy session with nurse: Patient says he is insecure. Feels his seventeen-year-old stepson can make decisions better than he can. Mentioned that he had had hopes of entering the ministry after graduating from high school but was called up for service because of the Korean War. Seems resentful toward God about this. Seems to have a very rigid conscience and his guilt feelings are high. He seems to be upset with himself about the least little thing he does wrong. This was pointed out to him. He seems to be quite depressed and will need to work hard while in treatment to maintain sobriety after he returns home. Has had some contact with AA and plans to return to AA when he goes home.

9/11
Therapy session with nurse: Patient talked about his previous involvement in youth work at church and with the Boy Scouts, stating that he would like to again become involved in these activities. He was reinforced in this plan. He talked about his feelings toward God. He said, "I guess I see Him more as a punishing God than a loving God. It was drummed into my head by my mother that if I did the wrong thing, Jesus wouldn't

love me." Differences between spirituality and religion were discussed further, and he was also referred to the chaplain, a suggestion which he seemed interested in following. His relationship with his mother was discussed—her possible influence on his perfectionist tendencies. When asked if he ever felt particularly happy about anything in his life, at first he didn't remember anything. Then he said that probably the happiest time was when he was given an award for being the best actor in a drama contest when in high school. He said he has had trouble with asthma all his life and could not go out for sports. He seems to have just realized that he has many resentments. He is showing a little insight at this time, but still is not thinking clearly at all times.

The patient took much responsibility in helping observe for DTs in a newly admitted patient. He seems to be doing a lot of thinking in his room. He does not seem to get in yet with other patients as "one of the group."

9/12
The patient is looking forward to the arrival of his wife and family. They went to church together and to the lake for a picnic.

Joint session with patient, wife, and nurse: Mrs. Alden seems fragile both physically and emotionally. She was encouraged to come to the treatment center for the last two weeks of Mr. Alden's treatment, which she plans to do. She discussed her feelings about the events precipitating Mr. Alden's present admission and also what led up to his admission in the mental hospital three years ago. She said that during Mr. Alden's previous hospitalizations she was told by the psychiatrist that sometime in his life he must have felt rejected by a loved one. The psychiatrist suggested then that Mrs. Alden show the patient as much love as she could—maybe more than in the past. He also suggested that she not yell so much at the children and Mr. Alden when they were doing things they shouldn't do. Because of this, Mrs. Alden said that for the last three years she has been keeping her angry feelings inside most of the time. She does look fairly depressed and like she needs someone to talk with. Mrs. Alden cried much of the session as she was expressing her pent-up feelings. Mr. Alden seemed to be looking out of the window during much of the session. When he was asked how he felt, he said "uncomfortable." He tended to minimize some of what Mrs. Alden was saying. It was pointed out to him that he needed to be honest. He seemed startled by this comment but said nothing.

9/13
Therapy session with nurse: Mr. Alden seemed very anxious for the therapy session today. He said that he had done a lot of thinking since

the joint session with his wife. Regarding his being told to get honest, he stated, "I thought I had been, but guess I haven't. I have been blaming Carol a lot for things that go wrong. I blamed Carol for a long time that we had to move in from the ranch because of her health." He mentioned that he learned a lot about himself today from the psychologist's lecture about defense mechanisms used by alcoholics. He mentioned his inferiority feelings. He says he has been told many times that if he would just be his real self, he would be a great guy; but he never could see that he was not being his real self. Now he is beginning to see that he has been setting up unrealistic expectations for himself. He seems to be seeing some of his "berserk" behavior when he is drinking and Carol expresses her anger at him. This needs to be discussed further. He says that he finds it difficult to talk about the things that are "bad" about him, but he knows that this is good for him in the long run. He said he felt better at the end of the therapy session than before. He plans to contact the chaplain and the AA counselor. He seemed to be sincere and to gain some insight in the session today.

9/14
Mr. Alden went to the AA meeting in town. He seemed to be quite interested in going to the meeting and encouraged other patients to go.

9/16
Mr. Alden conducted the 6 P.M. meeting. (Each patient and spouse in treatment takes his turn at conducting a one-hour evening meeting with patients.) He began with an autobiography. He seemed nervous, especially when he mentioned his wife having to go to work and his feeling "no good—depressed—nobody needed him." He could not look at the group for a while. The most pertinent remarks seemed to center around his feelings of unworth, guilt, and "no one cares"—especially his wife. He stated that he is a religious man with no spirituality. When the group began asking questions, Mr. Alden seemed to relax, but did get a little upset when he mentioned being an "introvert" and explained what he meant. By the end of the hour, he seemed very relaxed and reported that he felt good.

His minister was here during the meeting and Mr. Alden talked with him afterward.

Later in the evening, he played Scrabble with other patients and the nurse. He appeared quite relaxed. He mentioned he was pleased that his minister had come to the meeting.

9/19
The patient was mixing with different groups of patients most of the evening. He did not go bowling this evening because of a sore knee from

playing volley ball. He talked about how much he enjoyed church this morning, stating that he is probably in a better frame of mind this week than he has been for a long time.

Mrs. Alden and the children are visiting. Mr. and Mrs. Alden and the children played croquet, then went for a ride. The whole family seemed to be in good spirits.

9/20

Therapy session with nurse: Mr. Alden seems to be feeling better and making good progress. He has taken good action in talking with the chaplain and his own minister. He is now working on his fourth step of AA. He plans to take his fifth step with the chaplain in a few days. He also talked with the AA counselor, which he had been avoiding doing. He feels better since he has talked with him. Mrs. Alden had planned to come today for a joint counseling session but was unable to come. Mr. Alden said that the first time his wife came to visit, he did not particularly want her to come because he was afraid she would take some of the attention away from him. He said that this is the way he has been, in wanting to be more important than her at parties and other activities in which they have participated together. However, today he feels disappointed that she was not able to come. He says that this is a real change for him and that he is feeling closer to his wife than before. It was also pointed out that he seems to be feeling more secure with himself.

The patient was up until 1 A.M. talking with a new patient.

9/21

Note from chaplain: Mr. Alden took his fifth step today. Very good. He faced himself well and showed good insight.

In the evening, a friend of the patient visited and went to AA with him.

9/24

Mr. Alden played volley ball, then watched TV with other patients. He appears relaxed. Mrs. Alden has arrived for her week in treatment and has started her psychological testing.

9/26

Mr. Alden's "Hot Seat" was today. (During the Hot Seat, staff and patients write out the patient's assets and liabilities and spend an hour discussing these with the patient.) During his Hot Seat, Mr. Alden talked some about his experiences in the Navy. He responded quite well and was pleased with comments of other patients. He had difficulty accepting his assets.

MR. ALDEN'S HOT SEAT
(INCLUDING SOME OF HIS COMMENTS)

LIABILITIES	ASSETS
Could mix a bit more. ("Am afraid to approach people. Have to work on this.")	You are making a good effort and will no doubt see good results.
Easy does it. You aren't so bad as you seem to think. ("Too involved with myself.")	You are a very good gentleman. I've found you have a SINCERE and FRIENDLY personality. Your wife is one of your assets.
Don't try to rush the program. It will all come to you. ("I'm learning how to take it one step at a time.")	Seems to understand program fairly good. Keep up good work.
You don't seem to care to mix with others. ("Could be my inferiority feelings. I do like to be with people.")	Kind, sincere, and very interesting to talk with. Really is honest about his problems.
You are still thinking of the things that happened in the past.	Tim, you are a very likeable person and are trying very hard.
Needs more self-confidence. Needs to feel he has lots of self-worth.	You have a very good outlook on the future and are working hard to gain sobriety.
You need to work on your nerves.	You really know what the word ACTION means as you are showing it.
Can you see the need for daily living?	
Are you looking at one day at a time or too far ahead?	You are sincere and kind.
Still seems to be lacking some confidence, in handling his affairs. Do you really feel adequate in your job role and family role? ("Yes.")	Tim, I believe you are working hard and progressing well. You seem to be less nervous and really getting involved in the ACTION program.
Too perfectionistic. ("That's true, but I'm trying to do something about it.")	Has demonstrated what is meant by ACTION. You do seem to be making a good change—a result of your taking action to look at yourself honestly and do something about it.

9/27

Both Mr. and Mrs. Alden played volley ball with other patients. They also spent much of the evening visiting with another patient and his wife about their families and AA and Al-Anon.

9/28
Mrs. Alden conducted the 6 P.M. meeting. She told of her life and hard-ships. The group was helpful in making suggestions and would have been too quick to give her sympathy if the nurse had not intervened. She already appears to have found some answers to her problems. She seems open and willing to work problems out in the home. She discussed how she and Tim need to improve their communication. After the meeting, Tim went over and kissed her and told her how well she had done.

Mr. Alden went to AA and Mrs. Alden went to Al-Anon. Al-Anon is a group of spouses, family members, and friends of alcoholics who work together to help each other deal with their own problems.

9/30   12–2 A.M.
Mr. Alden sat with a newly admitted patient who may go into DTs.

Mr. Alden talked somewhat about last weekend when his wife and some friends from their church brought a picnic supper when they came to visit him. It was the regular meeting of their study group and the topic for the discussion was alcoholism. Mr. Alden talked with them about his experiences while in treatment and what he has gained. He seemed pleased that they all came and that he got to share his experiences.

10/1–2
Mr. and Mrs. Alden went home for the weekend. Upon returning, they said it had gone well.

10/4
Note from chaplain: Mrs. Alden took her fifth step today. Very good. She seems to be motivated to do anything to help herself, her husband, and their marriage.

Mr. Alden went to AA and Mrs. Alden went to Al-Anon.

10/5
Mrs. Alden had her Hot Seat, and handled it well. Mrs. Alden talked some about what the reactions of the children will be to Tim's changes. She is looking forward to a happier home life. She can see a big change—for the better—in Tim's behavior. She feels freer to talk with him and to express her feelings.

MRS. ALDEN'S HOT SEAT
(INCLUDING SOME OF HER COMMENTS)

LIABILITIES	ASSETS
You need to look at yourself more. You have not gotten rid of your problems yet. ("I have gotten a good start.")	Very nice person—enjoyable to talk to.
Don't let your children suffer from your childhood life. ("I have realized where I was wrong.")	Have made some very good progress for yourself. Good action and participation in the program.
I have the feeling you rule the roost at home. ("I *am* independent.")	Friendly and sincere.
Have you managed to "live for today" or are you still fearful of future? ("Goal for each day.")	Interested in others as well as herself. A very nice person. Realizes she can do better on her meal planning and housework. Seeks help.
Please stay out of the past more.	You seem to be trying very hard. Good work.
Past is past—leave it there. ("Past doesn't bother me anymore.")	She is a pleasant person to talk to.
Emotional control easily shaken up by current events. Talks freely of disliking cooking, planning meals. Does she know she can get help on this?	You have really shown progress and really seem happy. Good visitor.
You don't have it made yet. Think for yourself.	
Seems like a person that hasn't a temper but seems like she has a lot to learn about the program. ("I have a temper, but I am learning to count to 10.")	
Too dominating. ("I do end up doing things myself. I guess sometimes that make Tim less of a man.")	
Too independent. ("I'm kind of rebellious. Somebody tells me something for my own good and I do the opposite.")	
Do you feel you fully understand yourself at this point? ("No, but better than before.")	

10/7

Both Mr. and Mrs. Alden are looking forward to going home.

MY PLAN OF ACTION FOR MAINTAINING SOBRIETY (NOT NECESSARILY IN ORDER OF IMPORTANCE)

The following is what Mr. Alden wrote as his plan of action for maintaining sobriety when he returns home.

1. Daily meditations and an open "hot line" between God and myself.
2. Continuous communication between my wife and family, with the knowledge that I have my minister and treatment center, and AA members to fall back on if I feel something slipping.
3. Regular attendance in church.
4. Regular attendance in AA.
5. Periodic visits to the treatment center for counseling.
6. Redevelop an interest in my job, my family, and social life; also hobbies (not an overnight process—watch for "too much").
7. Further understanding and appreciation of myself as to the real me. Watch out for dishonesty and fantasy.
8. Living the AA program (all twelve steps—twenty-four hours a day).
9. Sharing and facing (with my wife and another person or persons connected) problems and situations as they arise. No procrastinations.
10. Carrying in my mind the slogan "Easy does it—but *do* it."
11. Unless unavoidable, try to stay away from drinking places such as pool halls, bars, etc. If unavoidable, face up to the situation with the strength I know I possess and understand to some extent.

DISCHARGE SUMMARY

Physical exam and lab tests: done.

Group counseling: attended all groups.

Individual counseling: nurse therapist, chaplain, AA counselor.

Other: individual sessions with wife, joint sessions with patient and wife, attended AA and church, fifth step, Hot Seat for both husband and wife, psychological testing interpreted for husband and wife.

Diagnostic impressions: Alcoholism.

Therapist's impressions: The patient has been motivated since his admission and has put much action into the program. Due to the honest effort he has made, there is a distinct change in patient's behavior and his feelings. He now feels confidence in himself, and this was certainly lacking when he was admitted. His wife was able to be in treatment the last two weeks the patient was in treatment, and the two of them working together has helped both of them. Both have been honest and have opened up communication channels which were not open previous to their treatment here. I feel that this couple has made an honest effort, and as their positive attitudes continue and as their actions continue, the chances for patient sobriety are excellent.

Prognosis: excellent.

FOLLOW-UP COUNSELING

11/2
Joint therapy session with nurse: Mr. and Mrs. Alden started the session by discussing a couple that they run around with in which the husband drinks heavily. They were concerned about his language around their children and how far to tolerate his unacceptable behavior. Then the patient brought up his wife's behavior of always being behind with housework, getting onto the children, and kidney trouble. The wife does seem to be very upset and cried during much of the session. The patient seemed to be understanding toward her but felt that she always had trouble with her kidneys whenever the pressure became too great. Thus, she would have an excuse to be behind with things and upset. The wife began to understand this and admitted that she feels very guilty if she ever sits down to rest. She feels sorry for herself when the rest of the family is together and she is in another room working. She seemed to get some understanding of her behavior but was still very upset at the close of the session because she wanted to know why she kept behaving this way. An individual appointment was set for November 18.

11/16
The wife is feeling fine, so she will not be here for the appointment November 18.

12/3
Joint therapy session with nurse: Mrs. Alden states she is having trouble feeling comfortable in church. Mr. Alden seems to be getting along fine. Both have been going weekly to AA. (There is no Al-Anon in their home town.)

Communication is improving but there is still some difficulty with finances. (They have been able to arrange for some Welfare help.)

PROGRESS NOTE FROM MR. ALDEN

This letter was received from Mr. Alden a year after his discharge. Mr. and Mrs. Alden had continued coming monthly for counseling at the treatment center.

Dear Friends:

Just a note to let you know what has been going on out here the last two weeks since we were down.

First of all, we are broker than anytime I remember. That is the main reason we didn't come down. We just plain don't have the long green to make the trip. Having to trade cars really cramped things for a few weeks, but am confident things will ease off in a couple of weeks.

I feel we are making some progress on our break in communication of the past few weeks. For a few days after our last counseling session things were a little bad, but as for myself, I realize now that the things that were bothering me then were for the most part just little petty things that didn't mean a whole heck of a lot.

I have been making an effort of doing at least one little job in connection with the house or family each evening after work instead of plopping my rear down on the sofa watching TV the rest of the night. This not only helps keep Carol off my back both verbally and silently (if you know what I mean) but gives me satisfaction in realizing accomplishments to do with helping around the house.

One attitude that I have been working on is the one where I figured Carol was the sole rudder of the house (ship). That her moods, attitudes, and habits were the only thing that could regulate the family moods and attitudes at home. After some deep thinking and experimenting, I am finding that not only is it unfair to Carol to put her in this position, but is also unfair to the kids and myself to have to depend on someone else's mood to regulate our own.

Carol has been working hard on the house. I still can't seem to get the drift of her plan of action and organization, but what the hell, I'll go along with most anything if it just gets the house clean.

Well, I got to go now. Will let Carol read this before I mail it. She might want to add some.

Regards to all,
Tim

STUDY GUIDE

1. What does the term "alcoholism" mean to you? How does one become an alcoholic?
2. Are the results of Tim's lab tests within normal limits?

3. Knowing Tim's medical history, which of the lab tests would you be particularly interested in? Why?
4. What is the nursing care if a patient develops alcoholic hallucinosis or delirium tremens?
5. What may be some reasons that Tim's first drink at age eighteen was a memorable one? (How does alcohol affect the central nervous system?)
6. How might the concepts of identity and identity confusion (developmental level—Erik Erickson) be useful in explaining the dynamics of Tim's alcoholism?
7. What clues do you have as to why Tim was so guilt-ridden? How did he express these feelings?
8. How did the treatment process affect Tim's perfectionism? Introversion?
9. What are the major defense mechanisms used by alcoholics? Give examples from the case and your actual experiences.
10. What could have triggered Tim's increase in drinking over the last few years? (What is one event you know took place in his life in the last few years?)
11. What particular adjustment problems did Tim's wife probably have
    a. before treatment?
    b. during treatment?
    c. after treatment?
12. What role did geography play in Tim's history and treatment?
13. What is *your* prognosis for Tim's future drinking behavior? Why?
14. Would you have included the Alden children in the treatment program? Specifically how?
15. What role might the community health nurse play in Tim's follow-up treatment? If you were making the referral, what information would you want the nurse to have?
16. What additional information, other than that presented in the case, would you have wanted about Tim and/or his wife?
17. What different approaches might you have taken in working with the Aldens?

SELECTED READINGS

W. C. Bier (ed.), *Problems in Addiction—Alcoholism and Narcotics*, Farthom University Press, New York, 1962.

E. M. Blum and R. H. Blum, *Alcoholism: Modern Psychological Approaches to Treatment*, Jossey-Bass, San Francisco, 1967.

M. E. Chafetz and H. W. Demone, Jr., *Alcoholism and Society*, Oxford University Press, New York, 1962.

S. Coopersmith, "Adaptive Reactions of Alcoholics and Non-alcoholics," *Quarterly Journal of Studies on Alcohol*, vol. 25, pp. 262–278, 1964.

J. Curlee, "Alcoholism and the Empty Nest," *Bulletin of the Menninger Clinic*, vol. 33, pp. 165–171, 1969.

Dilemma of the Alcoholic Marriage, Al-Anon Family Group Headquarters, Inc., New York, 1967.

E. X. Freed, "The Crucial Factor in Alcoholism," *American Journal of Nursing*, vol. 68, pp. 2614–2616, December 1968.

D. W. Goodwin, "Two Species of Alcoholic Blackout," *American Journal of Psychiatry*, June 1971, pp. 1665–1669.

C. H. Hartman, "A Structured Treatment Program for Alcoholics," *Hospital and Community Psychiatry*, vol. 22, pp. 35–38, June 1971.

M. Heyman, "Employer-Sponsored Programs for Problem Drinkers," *Social Casework*, vol. 52, pp. 547–552, November 1971.

J. K. Jackson, "The Adjustment of the Family to the Crisis of Alcoholism," *Quarterly Journal of Studies on Alcohol*, vol. 15, pp. 562–586, December 1954.

M. E. Kimmel, "Antabuse in a Clinic Program," *American Journal of Nursing*, vol. 71, pp. 1173–1175, June 1971.

B. Kinsey, "The Female Alcoholic," *A Social Psychological Study*, Charles C. Thomas, Springfield, Ill., 1966.

W. Knox, "Attitudes of Psychiatrists and Psychologists Toward Alcoholism," *American Journal of Psychiatry*, vol. 127, p. 111, June 1971.

M. Mann, *Marty Mann Answers Your Questions about Drinking and Alcoholism*, Holt, Rinehart and Winston, New York, 1970.

H. Mullan and I. Sanguiliano, *Alcoholism: Group Psychotherapy and Rehabilitation*, Charles C. Thomas, Springfield, Ill., 1966.

A. A. Parry, "Alcoholism," *American Journal of Nursing*, vol. 65, pp. 111–116, March 1965.

D. J. Pittman (ed.), *Alcoholism*, Charles C. Thomas, Springfield, Ill., 1959.

J. Pixley and J. Stiefel, "Group Therapy Designed to Meet the Need of the Alcoholic Wife," *Quarterly Journal of Studies on Alcohol*, vol. 24, pp. 304–314, 1963.

G. M. Price, "Alcoholism: Family, Community, and Nursing Problem," *American Journal of Nursing*, vol. 67, pp. 1022–1025, May 1967.

E. N. Scott, *Struggles in an Alcoholic Family*, Charles C Thomas, Springfield, Ill., 1970.

M. Victor, "Delirium," *Hospital Medicine*, vol. 6, pp. 116–129, March 1970.

R. F. Ward and L. A. Faillace, "The Alcoholic and His Helpers," *Quarterly Journal of Studies on Alcohol*, vol. 31, pp. 684–691, September 1970.

Mrs. Cox

thirty-eight years old

Abruptio Placenta/Acute

Betty L. Wilkerson and Rosemary Cannon Kilker

ADMISSION

Mrs. Cox, thirty-eight years old, Gravid v, thirty-eight weeks gestation, was admitted to the hospital having had no prenatal care. She complained of sharp, burning abdominal pain of approximately one to two hours' duration, with the passage of a small amount of dark blood per vagina.

NURSE'S ACTIONS

The nurse, the first person of the medical team to see this patient, was somewhat irate to think that Mrs. Cox had had no prenatal care, thus giving her no available baseline information to aid in her assessment. Multifaceted observations and care ensued simultaneously. While greeting Mrs. Cox and introducing herself, the nurse, by her self-assured manner, conveyed a feeling of security and relief. As the nurse assisted Mrs. Cox in disrobing and placing her on the examining table, through eye and tactile examination, the nurse assessed Mrs. Cox as to general appearance, color, and skin texture in relation to her condition, the feel of the uterus, and the present amount of bleeding. The nurse rapidly took the vital signs, took the fetal heart rate, and made a marking of the fundal height while also obtaining information concerning past health, other pregnancies, and the present pregnancy to this date.

The nurse's examination revealed the following findings: blood pressure 100/70, pulse 90, temperature 37°C, and fetal heart tones 140. The fundus measured 32 cm above the symphysis. The fetus was in the vertex position, but because of the tenderness and rigidity of the uterus, further palpation was not done.

MEDICAL TREATMENT

With this information at hand, the house officer was notified. While waiting for the physician to arrive, the nurse placed in readiness the crisis equipment and prepared Mrs. Cox for examination and fetal monitoring.

The physician verified the nurse's findings and ordered laboratory findings which revealed hemoglobin 12.0 g, hematocrit 36 percent, fibrinogen 300 mg/1000 ml, and proteinuria 1+.

A speculum examination revealed dark red blood oozing from the cervical os with the cervix dilated 2 cm. The cervix was 50 percent effaced and the presenting part was −1 station. Mrs. Cox had slight pedal edema accompanied with puffiness of the hands and face.

The physician's orders were as follows:

Nothing by mouth
Bedrest
Intake and output
Type and crossmatch 4 units of blood
100 ml of 5% glucose in water I.V. stat
Repeat fibrinogen level q. 2 h.
Attach fetal monitor after membranes are ruptured

Following the physician's evaluation, he apprised the family of Mrs. Cox's condition and the possible methods of treatment and possible problems that could be encountered with the baby. He also said that he or the nurse would keep them informed of Mrs. Cox's condition and that following the admission procedures, Mr. Cox could remain with his wife.

INTERVENTION

One hour post admission, the nurse's assessment was the same as originally noted except that the fundus now measured 34 cm above the symphysis. The blood pressure was 96/64, pulse 100, and fetal heart rate 132. The uterus was "woody." During this hour, Mr. Cox remained with his wife, but was asked to leave when Mrs. Cox was taken to the delivery room, where the membranes were ruptured artificially and the electrode and catheter were attached. Labor promptly ensued. Thirty minutes after rupturing the membranes, the fetal heart tones dropped to a rate of 100. Preparation was started for a stat cesarean section. However, before Mrs. Cox could be prepared for surgery, a matter of fifteen minutes, a stillborn male fetus was delivered spontaneously in a controlled unsterile procedure. Fetal resuscitation was to no avail.

The emotional support provided by the nurse during the crisis eliminated the necessity for sedation. This was accomplished by the nurse providing tactile reassurance to the mother, along with verbal explanation of what was taking place and directing Mrs. Cox in methods of relaxation.

Following delivery, the blood pressure dropped to 80/56 with a pulse of 116. A large retroplacental blood clot was expressed with a blood loss estimated at 2,500 cc. The physician ordered the first of four units of blood to be started I.V., and 50 mg Valium I.M. He then left to explain the situation to Mr. Cox.

After the nurse completed these orders, she prepared Mrs. Cox for a visit from her husband. In bringing Mr. Cox to the recovery room, the nurse asked Mr. Cox, "Would you like me to show the baby to you and your wife after she's rested awhile?" Mr. Cox's original response was, "What? What'd you say?" The nurse repeated her question. His response the second time was, "Do you think you should? Do you think she should see the baby?" The nurse stated, "Yes, the baby is a beautiful little boy and I believe it will be a comfort to you and Mrs. Cox to have seen him." Mr. Cox agreed that this seemed right, but asked for a little time to talk with his wife about it first.

Mrs. Cox remained in the recovery room for eight hours. By the end of this time, vital signs remained stable: blood pressure 110/80, and pulse 90. The uterus was firm and bleeding was minimal. The remainder of the postpartum course was uneventful other than for the emotional adjustment necessary in the loss of the baby.

STUDY GUIDE

1. What is abruptio placenta?
2. Discuss the etiology of abruptio placenta.
3. What are the two main types of bleeding in abruptio placenta?
4. Is abruptio placenta painful or painless?
5. When the abdomen of a patient having abruptio placenta is palpated, which characteristics vary from the "normal" gravid?
6. Which nursing assessments are necessary in the care of Mrs. Cox? Construct a hypothetical nursing care plan.
7. Discuss the nursing care of the mother who is placed on the fetal monitor.
8. What are some of the psychological implications of a labor patient who is having ultrasound monitoring?
9. How can the nurse effectively meet the special psychological needs of these patients?
10. Is a cesarean done if no fetal heart tones are heard?
11. Is the labor of a patient having abruptio placenta usually of long or short duration?
12. What is a couvelaire uterus? What is the treatment of a couvelaire uterus?
13. What is the usual prognosis for the fetus when the mother has the complication of abruptio placenta?
14. As Mrs. Cox has lost her baby, should she be placed postpartally on the maternity floor with other "normal mothers," on the maternity floor in a private room, or on a medical-surgical floor? Justify your answer.
15. Should Mr. and Mrs. Cox have been shown their stillborn child? Justify your answer.

16. Is it necessary for the nurse to help Mrs. Cox to cry?
17. Should Mrs. Cox be pushed through the grieving process?
18. As the nurse in the maternity area, how would you include Mr. Cox in this crisis of his wife and child?
19. Anticipating a difficult experience when arriving home, Mrs. Cox asks the nurse, "How will I be able to face the children? What will I tell them?" How would you respond to Mrs. Cox?

SELECTED READINGS

J. Beazley, "Inevitable Antepartum Hemorrhage," *Nursing Times*, August 12, 1971, pp. 985–987.

W. H. Blahd, *Nuclear Medicine*, 2nd ed., McGraw-Hill, New York, 1971, pp. 517–519.

L. L. Case, "Ultrasound Monitoring of Mother and Fetus," *American Journal of Nursing*, April 1972, pp. 725–727.

B. Drukker *et al.*, "Placental Localization," *American Journal of OB and GYN*, May 1, 1971, pp. 9–13.

E. Fitzpatrick *et al.*, *Maternity Nursing*, J. B. Lippincott, Philadelphia and Toronto, 1971, pp. 466–468, 485–489, 494–500, 505–506.

F. Goodrich, "Obstetric Hemorrhage," *American Journal of Nursing*, November 1962, pp. 96–97.

L. M. Hellman and J. Pritchard, *Williams Obstetrics*, 14th ed., Appleton-Century-Crofts, New York, 1971, pp. 609–635.

E. H. Hon, *An Introduction to Fetal Heart Rate Monitoring*, Harty Press, New Haven, Conn., 1971.

C. Lasater, "Electronic Monitoring of Mother and Fetus," *American Journal of Nursing*, April 1972, pp. 728–730.

J. Tucker, "Nursing Care in Obstetric Hemorrhage," *American Journal of Nursing*, November 1962, pp. 98–101.

J. Turbeville, "Nurse's Role in Hospital Care," *Hospital Topics*, June 1972, pp. 85–88, 103.

Mrs. Morgan
forty years old

Burned Patient/Acute
Carolyn Herrington Brose

Mrs. Morgan was aroused from her sleep by the persistent ringing of the alarm. As she rolled over to turn off the alarm, she looked at the gloomy winter sky. It was early—5 A.M.—and still very dark and very cold. She must get up and start her husband's breakfast. He had a great deal of work to do on their small farm before he left for his usual job in town. She also had a good many things to attend to before heading to Kansas City and her studies at the university research institute. Mrs. Morgan smiled to herself. It did seem silly to some that here she was, forty years old with five children and going to school! She wanted to complete her doctoral studies. What she was going to do after she got the degree she did not know for sure. One thing that she did know was that actually reaching that goal was the most important thing in her life right now. And why shouldn't it be! She had married young, had her family at a young age (three deliveries by cesarean section). The children were all independent now—Mike, the oldest, is in Vietnam. Mrs. Morgan's thoughts strayed from her self-defensive argument with herself—what is Mike doing now? Is he all right? Mrs. Morgan tried to shake the uneasy, empty feeling that always came when she thought of Mike's absence from home and his presence in a hostile environment.

Mr. Morgan arrived at the breakfast table. He did not kiss Mrs. Morgan, but only smiled and winked at her from his chair. It was the same as a kiss to Mrs. Morgan. After so many years of married life and hard work they did not seem to need the actual, demonstrative mode of expressing their deep love for one another. And, what with five children running about for so many years, it was hard to fight your way through the crowd sometimes. Mr. Morgan finished his breakfast and hurried on out to the barn to tend to the livestock before leaving for work. Mrs. Morgan looked at the clock; she just had time for one more cup of coffee and a cigarette before plunging into her tasks for the morning.

As she started to light her cigarette, Mrs. Morgan remembered that her lighter was almost empty. While filling the lighter, some lighter fluid splashed on the front of her flannel nightgown. Mrs. Morgan quickly brushed it off and thought little of the incident at the moment. She glanced at the clock again; she must hurry. Just time for that last cup of coffee. As she sat down at the table with her cup, she reached for a cigarette and her lighter.

Mr. Morgan had just left the barn when he heard the piercing scream. He stood for a moment, almost afraid to discover the cause and yet feeling he must get back to the house quicker than he could run. Panting from the run back to the house, Mr. Morgan burst into the kitchen. All he could see in his panic were the flames. "Marti, Marti!!" Somehow Mr. Morgan was able to extinguish the flames. Slowly he began to realize what had happened to his wife. Her gown had ignited when she lit her cigarette, she was badly burned, he had to get help!

The next several hours were almost nonexistent for both Mr. and Mrs. Morgan. Somehow during that time the ambulance came, the doctor came, and they found themselves entering the door of the hospital emergency room.

1. If you were in Mr. Morgan's position, what would you do for Mrs. Morgan?
    a. How would you extinguish the fire?
    b. Would you remove her clothing?
    c. Would you remove her jewelry, shoes?
    d. How and who would you summon for help?
    e. What would you do while waiting for help to arrive?
    f. What factors might affect Mr. and Mrs. Morgan's behavior at this point in time?
2. Mrs. Morgan's local medical doctor has called the hospital's emergency room to notify the staff that Mrs. Morgan was on her way.
    a. Why did the doctor call the emergency room?
    b. What thought should be given regarding transporting Mrs. Morgan at this time? Should any treatment be given before she is sent to the hospital?
    c. As the emergency room nurse in charge, what would you do in preparation for Mrs. Morgan's arrival and why? What information should you request from the doctor?

As the ambulance stops at the door, you have your first look at Mrs. Morgan. She is a small woman—probably only 5 feet, 1 inch at the most. She is very thin. Her eyes are open and you notice they are a beautiful steel blue color. You think to yourself—at least her face has not been burned. But, what lies beneath the sheet that engulfs her body?

"Mrs. Morgan, you're in the hospital. We are going to help you."

There is no response from Mrs. Morgan. Her gaze becomes blankly transfixed on the ceiling.

Your attention is drawn to Mr. Morgan. He has been directed to the admitting desk. You notice he has his hands grasped tightly together on the desk. His knuckles blanch white as he tries to respond to the clerk's questions.

"What is your wife's full name?"
    "Martha Diane Morgan."
"What is her birth date?"
    "November 20."
"What year?"
    "1930—I can't remember for sure . . ."
"How old is she?"
    "40."
"Has she ever been a patient here before?"

You notice Mr. Morgan's hands have begun to tremble. His chin is quivering as he tries to respond to the clerk's questions.

"Do you have any hospitalization insurance?"

Mr. Morgan breaks down into uncontrollable sobs as he shakes his head, "No" in response to the question.

3. What would you do for Mr. Morgan at this point in time? What behavior might be displayed and how will you intervene—or will you? Should you have intervened before this point in time?

EMERGENCY ROOM DATA

60% total body burn
2nd and 3rd degree burns on chest, and neck, right arm; small amount on left arm, back, abdomen and thighs.
Allergic to penicillin
Estimated body weight 105 pounds
No apparent inhalation of superheated air

TREATMENTS ORDERED

1. 1,000 cc lactated Ringers with #16 Jelco
2. #16 Foley with urimeter
3. 1,000 cc lactated Ringers with Erythromycin 500 mg I.V.
4. Demerol 50 mg I.V. and 50 mg I.M.
5. Plain tetanus toxoid 0.5 cc subq
6. Cutdown with 36 in. long catheter in right foot with lactated Ringers 1,000 cc
7. Dreft soap cleansing
8. Debridement
9. Sulfamylon cream applied to burn areas
10. Thoracic escharotomy

LAB RESULTS

1. W.B.C. 15,000
2. Hb. 16.8 g/100 ml

3. Hct. 47 ml/100 ml
4. Sp. Gr. 1.001
5. pH 5 (urine)
6. Na 140 meq/liter
7. K 4.0 meq/liter
8. Cl 106 meq/liter

TREATMENT PLANS

1. Admit to burn unit
2. N.P.O.
3. L arm I.V. 3,000 cc lactate Ringers 8 hr
4. R leg I.V. 1,000 cc Plasmanate; 2,000 cc D_5W
5. Erythromycin 500 mg q. 6 hr.
6. Digitoxin 0.4 mg x3 I.V.
7. Liver function studies
8. EKG
9. Chest x ray
10. Pulmonary care with O_2 tent and IPPB
11. Open wound care to all areas except hand

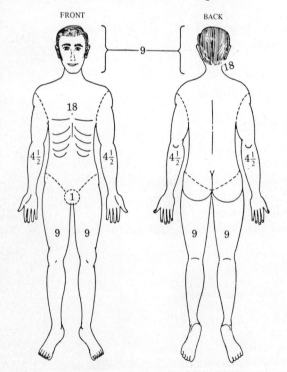

Summary	Percent
head	9
left arm	9
right arm	9
chest and abdomen	18
back and buttocks	18
left leg	18
right leg	18
G.U. area	1
	100

Estimation of Surface Area for Burns (Rules of Nines)

4. How are the burn depth and percentage calculated?
   a. Of what value is this calculation to therapy?
   b. When should this calculation be made?
   c. Does the Rule of Nines apply to adults and children alike? If not, what adjustments are necessary?
   d. How does the Rule of Nines compare with the Lund and Browder method of burn assessment?
5. What prognosis would you give for Mrs. Morgan at this moment? What factors did you take into consideration in determining her prognosis?
6. Why was a cutdown performed when an I.V. had already been started with a #16 Jelco?
7. Why was the Foley catheter inserted? Of what value would the urimeter be for Mrs. Morgan's therapy?
8. Why was the Demerol given as third degree burns are painless?
   a. Why was the Demerol given I.V. and I.M?
   b. What are the dangers of giving I.M. or subq injections to burned patients?
   c. Would you ever inject a medication into a burned area?
   d. Morphine is usually the drug of choice for burned patients. What are its advantages and disadvantages?
9. Why was tetanus toxoid administered?
   a. What is the difference between plain tetanus toxoid and aluminum phosphate tetanus toxoid?
   b. What is the normal dose of this drug for children and adults?
   c. Should Hypertet also have been given to this patient? Why?
10. Why was Dreft soap used for cleansing the burn wound? PhisoHex is usually used for cleaning most wounds.
11. What is debridement? What is its purpose?
12. What is Sulfamylon and why is it used?
    a. How is it applied?
    b. Is it painful to the patient?
    c. What are the advantages and disadvantages of Sulfamylon versus silver nitrate for treatment of burns?
13. What is escharotomy and why is it performed?
14. Were Mrs. Morgan's lab values within normal range? What does the statement "a shift to the left" imply?
15. Why was she made N.P.O.? Most burn patients are usually very thirsty.
16. Why was Mrs. Morgan to receive Erythromycin and Digitoxin?
17. Mrs. Morgan's I.V. fluids were calculated upon the Brooke formula. What is the rationale of this formula? Are there other formulas available to calculate fluid replacement for burn patients?
18. Why would Mrs. Morgan be placed in a O_2 tent with IPPB treatments also ordered? What respiratory complications might you observe for?

19. What would be your responsibilities to the patient and the attending staff while she is in the emergency room?
20. Mrs. Morgan was placed in a private room and in reverse isolation. Why was Mrs. Morgan placed in reverse isolation? How does reverse isolation differ from ordinary isolation procedures? Would you give any thought to sensory deprivation or sensory overload?
21. Mrs. Morgan is to be treated by the open method. What does this method consist of and how does it compare with closed methods of treatment?

HIGHLIGHTS FROM NOTES IN CHART

Feb. 1   5:30 A.M.
Patient climbed out of bed to bathroom pulling out both I.V.'s, Foley, O₂ tent. Restraints on all four extremities.

Feb. 2
Think patient is entering diuretic phase. No respiratory problems evident. Patient starting oral intake today.

Feb. 9
Low grade fever, erythema, edema to R hand, Seriously considering amputation. Hct. 40–30%. Will transfuse.

Feb. 10
Amputation of R arm.

Feb. 13
Febrile to 38.5°C. Seriously confused at ..mes.

Feb. 14
Febrile to 39.2°C. Cultures negative so far.

Feb. 20
To O.R. for debridement. Continues to be febrile during this period.

March 1
To O.R. for debridement and Split Thickness Skin Grafting (STSG). ST skin harvested from L thigh and leg. Applied to area of R arm stump.

March 10
To O.R. for Split Thickness Skin Grafting from leg to torso.

March 12
Spiking temp 38.5°C to 39.5°C. Over past 12 days wound cultures have been positive for Pseudomonas alrugrosa, urine cultures positive for *Candida albicans* and blood cultures have been positive for *Aspergillus fumigatis*. Urine was fluoresced last night. Questionably positive. Prognosis very guarded. Will continue with I.V.; hypercaloric, high protein, high carbohydrate, mineral and vitamins administered through jugular vein. Digitoxin, and Polymyxin B 400,000 units every 12 hours.

March 14
Positive fluorescence for Pseudomonas. Abdominal distention . . . due to impaction . . . removed.

March 16
Swine grafts applied.

March 20
Improving and temp decreasing. Has been lucid more frequently.

March 25
Spiking fever to 40. Essentially covered with either her skin or homografts. PROGNOSIS IS VERY POOR AGAIN. Blood cultures taken.

March 26
Overwhelming Candida growing from blood cultures. Infectious disease consult. Will start on Amptotericin B.

April 5
Has cellulitis L upper arm secondary to cutdown. Hot moist pack to site.

April 6
Temp coming down again. Patient looking better again.

April 12
To O.R. for Split Thickness Skin Grafting L leg, thigh, and hip (donor areas) applied to abdomen, neck, and chest.

April 26
To O.R. Split Thickness Skin Grafting taken R leg and L foot

ADMITTED FEBRUARY 1. DISCHARGED JUNE 1.

This is the first admission to this hospital for forty-year-old, white female who was brought into the emergency room following an acute burn.

History of present illness. On the early morning of the 1st of February, this patient sustained acute body burns following spilling cigarette lighter fluid over her gown.

Past medical history. Indicated that she had had five pregnancies and five deliveries with three cesarean sections. She then had a supracervical hysterectomy for fibroids. She has had blood transfusions without reactions. She has a history of moderate ethanol intake and is a chronic cigarette smoker.

Review of systems. Indicated that she had had a cigarette cough without hemoptysis and otherwise has been in fairly good health.

Physical exam. On admission to the emergency room showed the blood pressure of 120–130/70, pulse 116 to 125. There was second and third degree burns of the neck, shoulders, anterior chest wall, abdomen, anterior thighs, most all the right arm and hand and upper left arm and the left side of the back. This totalled about 60% of her body, of which at least half of it was thought to be third degree on admission.

Laboratory and x ray. Admission lab work hemoglobin was 17.2, hematocrit 50, W.B.C. 25,000 with a shift to the left. BUN, creatinine and electrolytes and proteins as well as liver function test were all within normal limits on admission. Numerous laboratory tests throughout her hospital course showed a hemoglobin as low as 8.8, and a hematocrit of 26 with a discharge hemoglobin of 11.5, hematocrit of 36 with a normal W.B.C. Urinalysis at the time of discharge showed 15–20 W.B.C.'s and a few bacteria. Electrolytes, proteins, and liver function tests were all normal prior to discharge.

Numerous creatinine clearance tests were essentially normal. Blood cultures throughout her course had shown Candida colonies innumerable. Urine culture intermittently showed Candida, Proteus, and wound cultures showed numerous bacteria including pseudomonas, coagulant positive staph, Proteus and Candida, x rays showed essentially no evidence of pneumonia. Electrocardiograms showed ischemia and digitalis effect.

Hospital course. Following admission through the emergency room the patient was washed down and debrided of loose and dead tissue and covered with Sulfamylon; she was put on a regimen of Sulfamylon application following washing with saline twice a day and given saline and plasma replacement per Brooke formula. She was digitalized and put on Erythromycin since she was allergic to penicillin. On 3/10 because of vascular compromise and infection in the right upper extremity, she had an amputation of the right upper extremity about the junction of the upper and middle third of the humerus. Throughout this course she ran fever intermittently. On 3/30 under general anesthetic she had debridement of her burns. She intermittently was changed and cleaned with Penthrane anesthetic on the ward and intermittently donor skin was applied to the areas which appeared ready for grafts. On 4/1 under general anesthetic she had further debridement of the scars with harvesting of Split Thickness Skin Grafting from her left thigh and leg and application of homografts on the rest of the areas that were ready for this.

Dressings were changed every day or every other day and homografts changed whenever available. On 4/10 under general anesthetic she had further Split Thickness Skin Grafting from her leg taken and placed mainly on her anterior trunk and at the same time a right internal jugular cutdown catheter was placed for the placement of hyperalimentation fluid therapy. Following this she continued to have spiking fever and pseudomonas and Candida were cultured from her urine and she was started on Polymixin B. She continued to have intermittent fever and dressing changes were performed nearly every day with either homografts or swine grafts applied to any areas that would appear to take grafts. The hyperalimentation program seemed to work very well and she began to improve and her temperature decreased. She was transfused periodically throughout this course. On the 25th of April she started spiking a very high fever and blood cultures were taken and her intravenous catheter (silastic) removed. These blood cultures showed overwhelming sepsis with Candida yeast and she was started on Amphotericin B. which was continued for a 21-day course. At this time she was nearly completely covered with either autografts or homografts but her course was precarious because of the fever and her sepsis and severe disorientation. On 5/2 she was found to have marked cellulitis to the left upper arm where the I.V. cutdown for the Amphotericin B. was and this was removed and she was started on another broad spectrum antibiotic for the cellulitis. Dressings continued to be changed nearly every day and the homograft again placed on any areas that were open. On 5/12 Split Thickness Skin grafts were taken from the left thigh and hip and applied to the abdomen and chest. These took very well and her course from then on improved. On 5/26 she was again grafted with Split Thickness Skin grafts from her right leg and foot and most of these took also. During this time she had rejection of some of the homografts on her chest and these were grafted with her own skin as it became available. By the middle of June she was started on ambulation again and treatment of her bilateral perineal palsies which probably resulted from positions necessary while she was being immobilized for grafting. She had developed moderately severe contracture at the neck and her stump never completely got covered over the bone. However, by 5/27 she had only very small areas on her right back and over her stump and her left neck that required coverage and it was felt that she could recover at home and return for further reconstructive surgery at a later date. Therefore, she was discharged on multiple vitamins and iron tablets and instructed in daily dressing changes and progressive ambulation. She will require revision of her stump and release of neck contractures at the very least as far as future reconstruction is concerned.

Final diagnosis. 60% total body burn including second and third degree burns of the chest and neck, right arm, right back, entire abdomen, and anterior of both thighs.

Mr. Morgan applied for welfare during March after discussing the projected costs of Mrs. Morgan's hospitalization. This was a very difficult move for this family as they are proud and hardworking people. They had always been self-supporting.

The County Welfare Department paid for Mrs. Morgan's hospital bill as well as for three pints of blood she had received. This amounted 'to a total of $12,593.05. Mr. and Mrs. Morgan still have to pay $375.00 for the remaining 15 pints of blood not covered by welfare as well as an orthopedic appliance for $61.00.

Mrs. Morgan was to return to this hospital for release of neck contractures in the fall, but sent a letter pleading to postpone the procedure until spring. She stated she was a coward and could not stand any more pain at this time.

Mrs. Morgan returned to the hospital the latter part of June to have her contracture release performed.

Her stay (fourteen days) was uneventful. Welfare once again paid her $715.00 hospital bill, but Mrs. Morgan had to pay $25.00 for a plastic neck collar.

Additional points for thought:

22. What is burn shock?
    a. Can it be prevented?
    b. How does it occur?
    c. How is it treated?
    d. How long does it last?
    e. What major fluid and electrolyte alterations occur during this stage?
23. What is the diuretic stage?
    a. Why does it occur?
    b. When does it occur?
    c. What major fluid and electrolyte alterations occur during this stage?
    d. Why does the development of digitalis intoxication become great during this stage?
24. What major electrolyte and metabolic changes occur because of burn injury? What effect do these changes have upon your nursing observations and care?
25. What is burn wound sepsis?
    a. How and why does it occur?
    b. Can it be prevented?
    c. What is the most often found organism in burn wound sepsis?

    d.   What are early clinical signs of sepsis? What is Woods lamp and why is it used?

26.   Why was Mrs. Morgan's arm amputated? How will you care for her stump? What response do you expect from Mrs. Morgan about her amputation?

27.   "A burned patient literally eats his way out of bed."
    a.   What nutritional requirements are necessary for the burned patient?
    b.   How can the nutritional requirements be met?
    c.   What is hyperalimentation fluid therapy?
    d.   What is paralytic ileus? How does it interfere with nutritional intake?
    e.   What is Curling's ulcer? How does it occur? How is it treated? Can it be prevented?
    f.   What is pseudo-diabetic syndrome? How might it occur in the burn patient?

28.   Mrs. Morgan had numerous grafting procedures performed.
    a.   What is the difference between autograft and homografts?
    b.   Why were swine grafts used on Mrs. Morgan?
    c.   What care must you give to the donor and/or recipient sites?

29.   What body image perception do you feel Mrs. Morgan would have of herself?

30.   Developmentally, what tasks of adult life do you feel she might be unable to complete?

31.   What differences are there between flame, scald, and electrical burns?

32.   What observations should be made on a patient who has received numerous blood transfusions?

ADDITIONAL POINTS TO CONSIDER WITH BURNED PATIENTS

1.   The donor site for skin grafting is equal to a second degree burn. Therefore, there is need to increase fluids and electrolytes to reach hemostasis during grafting.

2.   If mesh gauze is pulled from donor site too soon, the area will convert to a wound equal to a third degree burn. Gauze usually comes off after fourteen days.

3.   Hypothermia is a problem with scar tissue, especially in the O.R. A 40-watt bulb may be used to dry the graft as well as to conserve heat.

4.   Negroes, if grafted with white skin, will not convert to black color. The patient will have "pink" spots. There are make-ups available.

5.   There has been an increased incidence of malignancy in scar tissue occurring 10–20 years post burn.

6.   Blisters and pustules may be a problem for patients after recovery, as burn scars won't tolerate friction as normal skin will.

7. Sunburn also becomes a problem with patients after they have had grafting procedures.

8. Scars must be mature before reconstruction begins. Maturation usually takes 6–12 months. The scars become pale and flat as they mature.

9. Brooke Army Center is located in San Antonio, Texas. The Center has a 60-bed capacity and accepts military personnel or their dependents. The Center does no reconstructive work—provides only acute care. Patients usually arrive 24–48 hours post burn. Parents usually come with children. There are quarters for parents to stay in. The family does not have to pay for these accommodations. Military personnel continue to receive pay while staying with their child and are, therefore, not penalized by losing pay. Burned service men refer to themselves as "crispy critters."

10. Raw surfaces of burn should be separated (i.e., fingers) or they will grow together.

11. Electrical injury will produce muscle and bone injury. Thermal injury will usually produce skin and subcutaneous injury. Electrical burns are usually much more severe than they appear on the surface. If a person has suffered electrical burns, be sure to remove his shoes and examine the soles of his feet for burns . . . this is frequently the point of grounding.

12. Two types of splints are used with burned patients:
    a. Static Splint: nonmovable
    b. Dynamic Splint: movable (rubber bands, etc.)

13. Static splint must afford:
    a. maintenance of antideformity position
    b. distribute pressure evenly
    c. comfortable fit
    d. ease of application

14. CLEO makes assistive devices for activities of daily living.
    Cleo Aids
    3957 Mayfield Road
    Cleveland, Ohio 44121

15. Orthoplast (made by Johnson and Johnson Co.) is used to make splints. Splints are heated under running hot water and then molded for individual fit. Splints must be cleaned under cold water or in a gas autoclave.

16. Ear care: Second degree burns are very prone to chondritis. The patient may have to have cartilage removed. Do not allow the patient to have a pillow under his head if the ears have been burned.

17. The patient should begin turning as soon as possible after he is stabilized. If the patient will make himself "stiff as a log" it will make it easier to move him than if he is allowed to "sag."

18. If C.P.H. is given in small vessels, they will sclerose.

19. In the acute stage, if the head is kept dependent, the patient may have cerebral edema which may lead to convulsions.
20. If a patient becomes disoriented, the following should be considered:
    a. Is he toxic?
    b. Third degree burns: often can't tell where he is in space.
    c. Second degree burns: many sensations—all painful.
21. An increasing amount of skeletal traction is being employed to combat contraction formations.

SELECTED READINGS

Curtis Artz and John Moncrief, *The Treatment of Burns*, W. B. Saunders Company, Philadelphia, 1969.

Irene Beland, *Clinical Nursing: Pathophysiology and Psychosocial Approaches*, Macmillan, New York, 1970, pp. 880–908.

William S. Blakemore and William T. Fitts (eds.), *Management of the Injured Patient*, Harper & Row, New York, 1969, pp. 250–254.

John A. Boswick *et al.*, "The Critically Burned Patient: New, Simplified Approaches to Emergency Care and Rehabilitation," *Patient Care*, vol. 5, no. 10, September 15, 1971, pp. 72–136.

Frank C. DiVincenti *et al.*, "Inhalation Injuries," *The Journal of Trauma*, vol. 11, no. 2, February 1971, pp. 109–117.

B. W. Haynes, "Today's Challenge in Burn Therapy," *The Journal of Trauma*, vol. 10, no. 10, October 1970, pp. 811–815.

S. L. Fink, "Crisis and Motivation: A Theoretical Model," *Archives of Physical Medicine and Rehabilitation*, vol. 48, 1967, pp. 592–597.

D. Lavonne Jaeger, "Maintenance of Function of the Burn Patient," *Physical Therapy*, vol. 52, no. 6, June 1972, pp. 627–633.

Carl Jelenko, "Systemic Response to Burn Injury: A Survey of Some Current Concepts," *The Journal of Trauma*, vol. 10, no. 10, October 1970, pp. 877–884.

E. L. Lloyd and W. R. MacRae, "Respiratory Tract Damage in Burns," *British Journal of Anaesthesia*, vol. 43, no. 4, April 1971, pp. 365–379.

Barbara Minckley, "Expert Nursing Care for Burned Patients," *The American Journal of Nursing*, vol. 70, no. 9, September 1970, pp. 1888–1893.

John Moncrief and Basil Pruitt, "Electrical Injury," *Postgraduate Medicine*, vol. 48, no. 3, September 1970, pp. 189–194.

Tord Skoog, "Electrical Injuries," *The Journal of Trauma*, vol. 10, no. 10, October 1970, pp. 816–830.

Mrs. Winter
forty-two years old

Modified Radical Mastectomy/ Acute

Barbara Clancy

Breast cancer is the number one cause of death in women who die of cancer. Approximately 29,000 women and 250 men die of breast cancer every year. Between 65,000 and 75,000 new cases of breast cancer are diagnosed each year.

Although 90 percent of breast cancer is found by women themselves, only 65 percent of these women who find breast lesions present themselves to the physician.

The following is a case study to illustrate the physical and emotional nursing care involved for a patient and family experiencing a mutilating surgery of radical mastectomy.

GENERAL DESCRIPTION

Mrs. Winter, age forty-two, lives in a suburban two-story home with her husband and two teen-age children, a daughter sixteen and a son fourteen. She was admitted to the hospital for a breast biopsy and a possible mastectomy.

HEALTH HISTORY

Mrs. Winter considers herself and her family in "good health" both physically and emotionally. She stated that she discovered the lump in the left breast by accident during bathing. She was reluctant to be examined by her family physician; however, her daughter convinced her of the importance of an examination. Mrs. Winter had been hospitalized three years ago for removal of the gall bladder. There were no apparent problems during recovery.

Mrs. Winter has normal menstrual periods and has not experienced any physical or emotional signs of beginning menopause.

SOCIAL HISTORY

Mrs. Winter and her husband were married twenty-two years ago while both were pursuing a college education. Mrs. Winter taught elementary school until their daughter was born. Two years after the birth of their first child, a son was born. Mrs. Winter concentrated her energies on homemaking and family activities until both children were in school. When the children were ages eight and six, she returned to teaching school and is presently involved in part-time teaching in their neighborhood elementary school.

Mr. Winter is a manager for an advertising firm and has a Bachelor's degree in business administration. Although Mr. Winter has a responsible position involving extensive time and energy, the interrelationships of the entire family seem to be warm and supportive.

DAILY HABITS

Mrs. Winter arises early because all family members must arrive at work or school by 8:30 A.M. The children perform many household tasks and are responsible for certain duties. Mrs. Winter works two or three days a week as an elementary school teacher and this has not interfered with the home management.

Mr. and Mrs. Winter are involved in several social groups and enjoy many activities together.

NURSING ASSESSMENT

1. Nursing diagnosis
   a. Before surgery, the physical status of the patient was within normal limits except for lump in left breast
   b. Emotional status
      (1) Aware of high possibility of need for radical mastectomy
      (2) Demonstrated anxiety by tight facial expression, sweating palms, loss of appetite
      (3) Cried when husband was visiting
      (4) Asked questions about type of anesthesia used
2. Nursing plan—Preoperative
   a. Organize admission procedure in an individualized manner
   b. Administer physical skin preparation
   c. Include family in preoperative teaching
   d. Discuss immediate postoperative measures
      (1) turn, cough, hyperventilate
      (2) intravenous solutions
      (3) dressing and drainage equipment

e. Arrange for anesthetist to see patient and family
f. Allow patient to be able to discuss possible mastectomy and feelings and fears involved (discussion should not be forced on patient). Rehabilitation aspects can be introduced at this time if this would be helpful for specific patients.
g. Allow for family to express feelings and fears
h. Promote relaxation by administering nursing measures and sedative drugs at hour of sleep
i. Administer immediate preoperative nursing care
   (1) Operation permit signed
   (2) Safety measures
   (3) Notify family
   (4) Preoperative medication

Priorities

The priorities for nursing care will be based on the specific patient and family needs; however, the nurse should be aware of the fears and emotional significance involved in the alteration of body image when mutilation surgery is involved. The most important general nursing measures would be support and reassurance in a firm, compassionate manner.

SURGICAL TREATMENT

1. Modified radical mastectomy of left breast
   a. Removal of all breast tissue, nipple, and areola
   b. Removal of lymph in the axilla
   c. Muscles were left in place
2. Mrs. Winter was in surgery for 1½ hours. Nitrous oxide, oxygen, and Penthrane were the anesthetic agents used.
3. Drainage via hemovac apparatus was maintained.
4. Vital signs remained in the stable range throughout surgery: blood pressure 120/70, pulse 82.

POSTOPERATIVE MEDICAL ORDERS

1. Continue I.V. solutions for next 24 hr D_5RL 1,000 cc for next 8 hr, D_5W 1,000 cc for next 8 hr, and D_5RL 1,000 cc for last 8 hr of the 24-hr period. New solution order will be written if needed.
2. Demerol 75 mg q. 4 h. p.r.n.
3. Turn, cough, and hyperventilate.
4. Vital signs q. 15 min for 1 hr, then q. 1 h. for four times. When stable, every 4 hr for 2 days post-op.
5. Up on edge of bed in 6 hr.

6. Up in chair first post-op day.
7. Rehabilitation active exercises to begin first post-op day.
8. Maintain hemovac drainage for 24 hr.

POSTOPERATIVE NURSING INTERVENTION

1. Administer physical nursing care per medical orders.
2. Watch for drainage on bandages.
3. Provide for comfort measures, relieve pain, position.
4. Support patient in grieving process.
5. Give passive leg exercises to prevent thrombophlebitis.
6. Position arm to promote drainage.
7. Include husband and children in rehabilitative teaching.
8. Utilize a firm, consistent, and compassionate manner when beginning rehabilitation.
9. Teach self-care and safety practices.
10. Provide for cancer society representative to see patient in hospital if patient is so motivated.

HOSPITAL PROGRESS

Mrs. Winter was depressed after surgery, which was a normal reaction. Physical progress was good and she tolerated progressive arm and finger exercises.

On the fourth day after surgery, Mrs. Winter became quite discontented with the nursing care, the medical care, and the hospital in general. She demonstrated anger and asked, "Why me?" for the first time since hospitalization. Her family was upset with her reaction but understood her feelings. That evening she applied makeup, combed and brushed her hair, dressed, and went for a walk in the hall, on her own initiative.

On the fifth day, the pressure bandages were removed; however, she did not want to look at the scar. Later that evening she requested that the nurse remove the bandage so that she could see the scar.

On the sixth day after surgery a representative from the Cancer Society visited Mrs. Winter and showed her the different types of prostheses available.

Mrs. Winter was dismissed on the seventh postoperative day. Her family had been in attendance every day of her hospitalization. The special needs for Mrs. Winter had been discussed with the family by both medical and nursing personnel.

CONTINUITY OF CARE

1. Continued supportive and rehabilitative nursing care should be provided through a community health nursing referral.

2. Continued nursing care should be provided so that the progress and adjustment of the patient and family can be observed and evaluated.
3. Continued nursing care can provide supportive measures to help the patient and family meet their needs during the post-surgical period.

STUDY GUIDE

1. Review the seven cancer warning signals.
2. What kind of women are prone to develop breast cancer?
3. What are the various methods of diagnosing breast cancer?
4. Why are some women reluctant to seek medical care upon finding a lump in the breast?
5. What are some of the feelings of persons experiencing a mutilating surgery?
6. Review crisis theory. How can this knowledge be utilized to help a patient and the family during the rehabilitative process?
7. How can the loss of a breast affect a woman's feelings about sexuality? A husband's feelings about sexuality?
8. What are the signs of breast cancer?
9. What steps are involved in breast self-examination?
10. Describe the different types of breast surgery
   a. Lumpectomy
   b. Simple mastectomy
   c. Modified radical mastectomy
   d. Standard radical mastectomy
   e. Supraradical mastectomy
11. Review the preoperative teaching for a patient having a mastectomy.
12. How could the family be involved in preoperative teaching?
13. Describe the passive and active exercises during the postoperative period.
14. What specific safety factors are taught patients after a mastectomy?
15. What follow-up care (medical and nursing) should be provided the patient and family?
16. What type of resources are available from the Cancer Society?
17. Describe augmentation surgery after mastectomy. Are there any dangers?

SELECTED READINGS

D. Berry, "Support from Nursing Staff Helps Nurse–Patient Cope with Cancer," *Hospital Topics*, vol. 48, October 1970, p. 60.

H. Bronson, "The Nurse and Mutilation Reaction," *Bedside Nurse*, vol. 3, September 1970, p. 26.

"Breast Cancer," *Post-Graduate Medicine*, vol. 48, August 1970, p. 192.

"Breast Cancer: Detection, Management, Rehabilitation," *Journal of Practical Nursing,* vol. 21, May 1971, pp. 20–24.

M. Corbeil, "Nursing Process for a Patient with a Body Image Disturbance," *Nursing Clinics of North America,* vol. 6, March 1971, pp. 155–163.

J. B. Davis, "Subcutaneous Simple Mastectomies with Implantation of Mammary Prostheses," *Nebraska State Medical Journal,* vol. 55, December 1970, pp. 726–728.

H. Dillon, "The Woman Patient," *The Nursing Clinics of North America,* vol. 3, June 1968, p. 195.

G. Fitzpatrick, "Caring for the Patient with Cancer of the Breast," *Bedside Nurse,* Part 1, vol. 3, February 1970, p. 20.

G. Fitzpatrick, "Caring for the Patient with Cancer of the Breast," *Bedside Nurse,* Part 2, vol. 3, March 1970, p. 19.

C. A. Gribbons *et al.,* "Treatment for Advanced Breast Carcinoma," *American Journal of Nursing,* vol. 72, April 1972, pp. 678–682.

H. C. Harrell, "To Lose a Breast," *American Journal of Nursing,* vol. 72, April 1972, pp. 676–677.

G. Letterman *et al.,* "Reconstruction of the Breast Following Sub Q Simple Mastectomy," *Journal of the American Medical Women's Association,* vol. 23, October 1968, pp. 911–915.

J. R. Lewis, Jr., "Reconstruction of the Breasts," *Surgical Clinics of North America,* vol. 51, April 1971, pp. 453–469.

P. Mayo and N. Wilkey, "Prevention of Cancer of the Breast and Cervix," *The Nursing Clinics of North America,* vol. 3, June 1968, pp. 229–241.

B. Meyer, "The Psychological Effects of Mutilating Operations," *Medical Insight,* vol. 2, September 1970, p. 82.

N. C. Nelson, "Discusses Methods of Diagnosis, Treatment, of Breast Cancer," *Hospital Topics,* vol. 49, pp. 79–80, June 1971.

M. L. Owen, "Special Care for the Patient Who Has a Breast Biopsy or Mastectomy," *Nursing Clinics of North America,* June 1972, pp. 373–382.

M. M. Ravitch, "Alternatives to Halstedian Radical Mastectomy," *Medical Topics,* vol. 99, April 1971, pp. 119–120.

R. K. Snyderman *et al.,* "Reconstruction of the Female Breast Following Radical Mastectomy," *Plastic Reconstruction Surgery,* vol. 47, June 1971, pp. 565–567.

W. D. Shorey, "Carcinoma in Situ of the Breast," *Surgical Clinics of North America,* vol. 51, February 1971, pp. 75–82.

Mrs. Williams
forty-five years old

Cancer of the Cervix/Acute
Rosemary Cannon Kilker and Betty L. Wilkerson

ADMISSION

Mrs. Williams is a forty-five-year-old mother of three teen-age children. She was admitted for irregular and heavy vaginal bleeding. The nurse entered Mrs. Williams's room to begin her assessment.

Nurse: "Good afternoon Mrs. Williams. I'm Martha Ross, a staff nurse on this unit. I want to help you with the admission procedure and ask some questions for our records."

Mrs. Williams: "I'm so glad you've come in just now. I'm so worried and frightened."

Miss Ross placed her hand on the patient's hand. In so doing, she noticed the texture of the skin, the trembling of Mrs. Williams's arm, and the moisture of her hand. She then proceeded to talk with Mrs. Williams to help her to relax while obtaining vital signs, weight, blood pressure, and a urine specimen. These assessments revealed a pale, forty-five-year-old, 5 foot 4 inch tall lady, moderately obese, and weighing 71.8 kg. Her blood pressure was 140/90, pulse rate 88, and temperature 37°C. The nurse learned that Mrs. Williams was a housewife and has three children: John, age nineteen; Chelsea, age sixteen; and Don, age fourteen. Mr. Williams is a certified public accountant. The family resides in a middle-class suburb. Mrs. Williams's mother and father are living and well. She has no siblings. Mrs. Williams is quite active in community and church affairs.

NURSING HISTORY

The nursing history revealed that at the age of thirty Mrs. Williams was told that she had fibroid tumors which should be watched. At the age of thirty-five her menstrual flow became twice as heavy. However, she had no other symptoms at this time. There is no history of weight change and all Papanicolaou smears have been negative. A dilatation and currettage was done at the age of thirty-seven and again at the age of forty because of intermenstrual bleeding. No malignancy was reported. Mrs. Williams has taken iron for years because of anemia due to excessive menstrual bleeding. When asked about other bleeding, Mrs. Williams said that for the past six months she has had some bleeding after intercourse. Her last menstrual period was one week before the hospital admission. Mrs. Williams said that hysterectomies "run in the family." Her mother and her aunt had hysterectomies when they were in their forties.

After receiving this information, Miss Ross explained that the physician would be in shortly to do a complete medical examination, including a pelvic, and to ask additional questions. Mrs. Williams immediately requested that she be able to take a douche and wash again. Miss Ross said, "No, I understand how you feel about being extra clean for a pelvic; however, washing and douching immediately before may alter the lab results and the doctor's observations of your tissues."

MEDICAL EXAMINATION

Upon medical examination, pertinent physical findings were limited to the abdomen and pelvis. There was a well-healed McBurney's scar and a firm, irregular suprapubic mass that rose to 5 cm above the symphysis. It was slightly tender and movable. Pelvic examination revealed a parous outlet with good support. The patient had a thick, brownish-yellow discharge. A cervical lesion of approximately 3 cm was seen. A Papanicolaou smear and punch biopsies were obtained. The uterus was in mid-position and irregular. No adnexal masses were palpable. There was thickening of the uterosacral ligament on the right and some nodularity was felt.

The laboratory reports were: The Papanicolaou smear was negative, but the biopsies showed squamous cell carcinoma, grade three. Two methods are available for the treatment of this type of carcinoma: radiation or radical surgery. In neither method is the prognosis good due to the extensive lesion.

When the physician discussed Mrs. Williams's condition with her and her husband, the nurse was present. With his advice, radiation therapy was the treatment chosen by Mr. and Mrs. Williams. After the physician left, Miss Ross remained with the couple to see if she could help them and answer any unasked questions. Miss Ross left after a short time, permitting Mr. and Mrs. Williams to work through their feelings.

NURSE'S ACTIONS

When the nurse entered the room later, Mrs. Williams began to review all the physician had told her. She would ask, "Now, that is what he said, wasn't it? It's hard for me to remember everything." She also asked, "There's no way the tests could be wrong, is there?" The nurse understood that she was still having problems accepting the diagnosis, but she explained how the specimens were labeled and the reports obtained. It was not long until Mrs. Williams requested the nurse to tell her more about radiation—how painful it really was, and whether it was true that she could not have any visitors.

Miss Ross relieved her fears as much as possible and reassured her that the inactivity and backache were the most bothersome complaints while the radium was inserted. She also explained that visitors and staff were allowed, but only for short periods of time due to the radiation effects from which they would not be protected.

The next morning, Mrs. Williams was taken to surgery for radium insertion. The physician outlined the medical treatment again, and the radiation precautions were reexplained. A Foley catheter was inserted, and it was explained that this was to keep her bladder empty to prevent excessive radiation of the bladder, which is in close proximity to the radium. The low residue diet, Geiger counter checking, examination of linens, and exact visiting restrictions were again discussed.

Mrs. Williams needed visual, tactile, and verbal communication during radiation therapy. She became concerned if she would possibly be "radioactive" following the removal of the radium. Miss Ross explained that this was not possible. She sincerely appreciated the staff stopping at the doorway during her "wakeful" hours, to say just a few words now and then. She felt that her real needs were minimal, but that the time passed slowly. Seventy-two hours later, Miss Ross accompanied Mrs. Williams to have the radium removed. Following a bath and medicated douches, Mrs. Williams was up, walking about in her room, and looking forward to going home.

Before dismissal, Miss Ross and the physician discussed with the Williams the absence of any radioactivity now, the importance of continued medical guidance, and the resumption of household, social, and sexual activities.

STUDY GUIDE

1. Discuss the well-recognized predisposing factors of uterine fibroids.
2. What emotional overlay can be caused by fibroids?
3. What are some of the necessary points that must be included in the nurse's counseling with the patient having bleeding fibroids?
4. With Mrs. Williams's case in mind, how would you answer the question, "Why bother with Pap smears?"
5. What anticipated benefit is derived from estrogen-progesterone therapy?
6. Discuss squamous cell carcinoma of the cervix in regard to etiology, metastasis, and symptoms.
7. What are the anticipated emotional problems of Mr. and Mrs. Williams due to the diagnosis?

8. In discussing surgery versus radiation treatment, how can the nurse respond to the Williams's question, "What choice would you make?"
9. What teaching is necessary to prepare Mr. and Mrs. Williams for radiation therapy?
10. What effects will radiation therapy have on the neoplastic sites and the surrounding tissue?

SELECTED READINGS

American Cancer Society, Inc., *A Cancer Source Book for Nurses*, 1968.

M. Barnett, "The Nature of Radiation and Its Effect on Man," *Nursing Clinics of North America*, no. 1, March 1967, pp. 11–22.

D. Berry, "Support from Nursing Staff Helps Nurse–Patient Cope with Cancer," *Hospital Topics*, October 1970, pp. 60–62.

E. H. Boeker, "The Nurse in Radiation Protection," *Nursing Clinics of North America*, no. 1, March 1967, pp. 23–34.

J. Brewer *et al.*, *Gynecologic Nursing*, C. V. Mosby, St. Louis, 1966.

D. Buchler *et al.*, "Radiation Reactions in Cervical Cancer Therapy," *American Journal of OB and GYN*, November 15, 1971, pp. 745–750.

M. Davis, "Patients in Limbo," *American Journal of Nursing*, April 1966, pp. 46–48.

H. Green, Jr., *Gynecology—Essentials of Clinical Practice*, Little, Brown, Boston, 1971, pp. 301–331.

R. Hilkemeyer, "Nursing Care in Radium Therapy," *Nursing Clinics of North America*, no. 1, March 1967, pp. 83–96.

E. Hoffman, "Don't Give Up on Me," *American Journal of Nursing*, January 1971, pp. 60–62.

S. Klagsbrun, "Communications in the Treatment of Cancer," *American Journal of Nursing*, May 1971, pp. 944–948.

E. Kubler-Ross, *On Death and Dying*, Macmillan, New York, 1969.

N. Miller and H. Avery, *Gynecology and Gynecologic Nursing*, W. B. Saunders, Philadelphia and London, 1965.

E. Novak *et al.*, *Novak's Textbook of Gynecology*, Williams & Wilkins, Baltimore, 1970, chaps. 12, 16.

J. W. Roddick, Jr. *et al.*, "Treatment of Cervical Cancer," *American Journal of OB and GYN*, March 1, 1971, pp. 754–759.

P. S. Rummerfield and M. J. Rummerfield, "What You Should Know about Radiation Hazards," *American Journal of Nursing*, April 1970, pp. 780–786.

J. Shepardson, "A Team Approach to the Patient with Cancer," *American Journal of Nursing*, March 1972, pp. 488–491.

Van Nagell *et al.*, "The Staging of Cervical Cancer: Inevitable Discrepancies Between Clinical Staging and Pathologic Findings," *American Journal of OB and GYN*, August 1, 1971, pp. 973–978.

A. Verwoerdt, "Communication with the Fatally Ill," *Southern Medical Journal*, 1964, pp. 787–793.

E. Walker, "Responsibilities of the Hospital Nurse in the Clinical Use of Radiation," *Nursing Clinics of North America*, no. 1, March 1967, pp. 35–48.

J. Walter, *Cancer and Radiotherapy: A Short Guide for Nurses and Medical Students*, J. & A. Churchill, London, 1971, pp. 133–144.

Mrs. Carlton
forty-eight years old

Involutional Depression/Acute
Elaine Darst

NURSING HISTORY

Mrs. Carlton is a forty-eight-year-old married woman admitted to a state hospital in January 1969, with the diagnosis of involutional depression. She is a short slender lady of small build, neatly dressed, her hair well-groomed, and her modest amount of makeup neatly applied. She resides in a small, southern rural community with her husband and one son, aged fourteen. Their income depends on the business from a garage that her husband owns. Their house was described by Mrs. Carlton as small and not well decorated as compared to the homes of her friends. She frequently mentioned the remodeling process in which they were involved, which included major carpentry work on the bathroom. Mrs. Carlton did not work outside the home, and described her major activities as housekeeping and some church and club activities.

This admission to the hospital was her first, previous to which she had been seen by a private psychiatrist for several months. During the time she had seen the private psychiatrist, she reported that her anxiety and depression continued to increase until hospitalization was recommended. When she entered the hospital, her main complaints were nervousness and depression. The nervousness was manifested by her inability to sit or stand still, by her constant picking of her fingernails and surrounding skin, by her alternating jerky body movements and rigid straight posture, and by her fidgeting. Her depression was evident by her sad facial expression, lack of spontaneity, monotone voice, lack of interest in her usual activities, withdrawal from important people in her life, and her reports of feeling like crying.

Mrs. Carlton dated the beginning of her illness to June 1968, saying this is when she began to feel depressed. However, her husband had noticed it earlier. During June 1968 she dropped out of her church circle (a women's organization), which she had regularly attended. She and her husband also discontinued square dancing, although this was due to the husband's desire. Square dancing had been an enjoyable endeavor for Mrs. Carlton. At this time, she felt like staying home all the time, although she did continue to attend Moose Club and American Legion Auxiliary up until hospitalization. Her interest in her activities at home also decreased. She no longer enjoyed cooking, and found that she had no desire or energy for her usual routine of housework. Mrs. Carlton also recalled that in June 1968, her son broke his arm, but she did not attribute her illness to this event.

She believed that her illness might have been due to menopause, which began about one year prior to admission. She also recalled the beginning of many fears about the time menopause began—fears about the future, especially about income, fears about illness, and indirectly, fears of death. She verbalized fears about hemorrhaging during menopause and the possibility of not being able to get help for it quickly enough. Included in her ideas about menopause was a fear of becoming pregnant again. Her fears of illness were accentuated by her identification with her father's physical disabilities. So, for Mrs. Carlton, the future seemed bleak, as she imagined illness for herself and her husband, a decrease in income, an inability to continue gratifying activities, and in general, little satisfaction from growing older.

In describing her background, Mrs. Carlton reported the following information. She was born the youngest of three children in a rural southern community. She stated that her parents had not wanted a third child, although they did not openly reject her. Her father had been a farmer, but had to retire while the patient was very young because of his numerous physical disabilities. He was a strict father who would not allow her to date as a teenager. However, her mother encouraged her dating, and the two of them deceived her father by making up alibis when she dated. Her father died when the patient was age seventeen. She stated that she was always closer to her mother than her father. Her relationship to her siblings, one brother and one sister, both over four years older than she, was that of the young "spoiled" baby of the family. She always felt left out by them because she was younger.

Of her school years, she remembered teachers telling her she was spoiled and had her own way too much. She also remembered having an explosive temper, for which everyone chastised her. At this time, she had fears of getting out of control which she verbalized as the impulse and fear that she would throw objects at people with whom she was angry. After her adolescence she did not remember having a problem with her temper.

After graduating from high school, she lived at home with her mother and worked a short time in a national youth work program organized during the World War II years. She had desired to marry a young man she was dating when she was about age seventeen, but her mother opposed this marriage, and he left for the Army. She states that it is better that she waited. At age twenty-six (in 1947), she married her present husband. She said nothing about courtship or about her emotional involvement with him. For a while, she worked in her husband's filling station doing bookkeeping. After he obtained a garage, she stopped working for him, and had not helped in the business since, although he had asked for her help in recent years. During the major part of her married life, she had been a housewife, and her meticulous housekeeping was a source of irritation to her husband.

Eight and one-half years after she was married, she gave birth to a son. She stated that they did not want the child, and after he was born, she became very nervous and preoccupied with fears of his dying. She had no professional help then. When asked if she had problems with her son at that time, she reported none. In her description of him, she stated he was much like her— quiet and shy. He did poorly in school, and she was afraid of his failing. He played with children younger than himself and was interested in model cars and other things. Mrs. Carlton also feared that her son would not be a successful adult and that she would continue to have to care for him.

Two years after her son was born (1957), her mother died. She said she missed her mother, but had become quite close to her mother-in-law. Six years ago, her mother-in-law went to a Masonic retirement home in a large town about two hundred miles away. After this, she became closer to her older sister as one on which to depend. Her life pattern had been characterized by dependence on these figures and on her husband. Ambivalence about those she depended on was evident in some of her behavior. For example, she did not want her sister to visit her at the hospital, even though she was close to her. Also, when the subject of weekend visits to her home was discussed, she expressed a desire to go home, but said she could not because the bathroom remodeling was not finished, which made her nervous. In working with her, the nurse noted ambivalence in the nurse–patient relationship. Mrs. Carlton would approach the nurse, then walk away; would begin to speak with the nurse, then tell the nurse to talk with someone else.

OTHER SIGNIFICANT DATA

Rest and sleep patterns. Early in her hospitalization, Mrs. Carlton went to bed at 6 P.M., but did not sleep until she had sleeping medication. After this, she slept the entire night.

Elimination. She took laxatives regularly.

Eating. She was always concerned about her weight, thinking she ate too much. At one time, she made an effort to lose weight (later in hospitalization).

Activity and recreation. She enjoyed square dancing, spectator sports, and club activities. She played basketball at the hospital, but not aggressively.

Interpersonal and communicative patterns. When she tried to sit, her body looked rigid; her legs were never crossed, but were close together and stiff. She had intermittent eye contact, but usually had her eyes lowered. Her eyes showed expressions of fear, submissiveness, and anxiety. She spoke in a quiet voice which wavered at times and had very little inflection. She seldom talked spontaneously, but always answered questions, usually as briefly as possible. Many times her answer was, "I don't know," or "I can't remember." (This was predominant at the beginning of her hospitalization.)

Temperament. She was anxious, shy and docile, and controlled, exhibiting emotions in a very limited way.

Dependency and independency patterns. She seemed to cling to one friend she had at the beginning of her hospitalization, asking this friend to make many decisions for her, e.g., which direction to walk. There was a pattern of dependency throughout her life. She recognized her dependency on her husband. She always took the passive role in this relationship, as in others. For example, she asked her husband to speak with the doctor rather than doing it herself.

Mrs. Carlton remained at the hospital almost five months. She was maintained on Tofranil 25 mg four times a day, and Thorazine 100 mg three times a day. During her stay, she changed from being very anxious, withdrawn, and depressed to being more spontaneous, energetic, and happy. She returned to her state of normal functioning. At her discharge in mid-April, plans were made for her to be maintained on her medication and supervised by her hometown physician. She would return to the hospital for at least one outpatient visit for evaluation of her progress.

NURSING CARE PLAN FOR MRS. CARLTON

Problem One: Anxiety

Mrs. Carlton manifested a great deal of anxiety, as described in the nursing history. In the early part of the nurse–patient relationship, she had to walk constantly. She could not sit for more than a few seconds. Her attention span was short. She also verbalized the fact that she felt nervous.

The compulsive character structure that Mrs. Carlton had maintained previous to her illness had broken down. At this time, her ego no longer had the strength to maintain this way of functioning and thus bind tension. Consequently, the anxiety was more free-floating and discharged in the way described.

When the nurse first approached Mrs. Carlton, introductions were made and Mrs. Carlton stood for a bit picking her nails, lifting her feet up and down, looking worried. Then she said she could not talk—that the nurse should find someone else—and walked away. The second approach made by the nurse was with more persistence, and the patient was requested to sit and talk. It soon became evident that Mrs. Carlton could not sit, as she stood up and began to terminate the contact. It was then the nurse realized some flexibility was needed in dealing with this anxiety, so she suggested a walk. This proved to be the best activity for discharging some anxiety, while engaged in conversation. Gradually the periods of time in which the nurse and patient spent walking decreased, and the patient was able to tolerate increased periods of sitting. This was accompanied by an ability to also attend other functions, such as church, without having to leave.

At the beginning of the relationship, the nurse tended to ask numerous questions of the patient. As questions increased, the patient's responses decreased, and communication seemed to halt. The nurse then needed to explore the interaction, including her feelings, to discover the block in communication. The nurse's questioning was a result of her own anxiety, stemming from two sources. The patient's anxiety was communicated to the nurse, which was added to the nurse's own original anxiety created by her desire to prove herself an effective therapist for professors in graduate school. Understanding that the questioning led to little response, the nurse changed her approach, decreasing the questions and helping Mrs. Carlton feel as comfortable as possible by accepting her in a nonjudgmental way. Added to the walking and decreased questions, the nurse began focusing on topics easier for Mrs. Carlton to handle when her nonverbal behavior indicated an increase in anxiety. All these things had the effect of decreasing the anxiety in both the nurse and the patient, and the relationship began to develop more naturally and easily for both.

A major approach used in dealing with the anxiety was to encourage verbalization about those things that caused an increase in anxiety, i.e., angry feelings. The nurse originally placed much emphasis on controlling the anxiety, with Mrs. Carlton receiving praise for sitting for longer periods of time. Mrs. Carlton thus began to report more about how she had sat through some meetings, rather than discussing her feelings. Her anxious behavior still continued while she was with the nurse. At this point the nurse began to give more praise for the expression of feelings and less for control of anxious behavior. This reinforcement for discussing feelings and situations causing anxiety was necessary since Mrs. Carlton avoided those topics and openly said she did not like discussing them.

Another productive approach to Mrs. Carlton was helping her rebuild her compulsive personality structure. Without prompting from the nurse, Mrs. Carlton did this on her own, devising a schedule for herself. The nurse was delighted and continued to encourage her to do this at the hospital as well as during her weekends at home. Near the end of her hospitalization, Mrs. Carlton said that her husband had previously asked her to work in his garage, doing such things as keeping supplies in order. The nurse later asked if she had talked with her husband about doing this after discharge. She said "no," that she did not think she would do it. However, on discharge day, she said she had mentioned it to her husband and might go to work. The nurse was pleased, saying enthusiastically, "Good, I think you will do an excellent job with that. You like to keep things neat and orderly, which should be a big help in a garage." Mrs. Carlton's eyes twinkled, showing how pleased she was with herself. Consequently, the compulsive activities were encouraged as a discharge recommendation also.

Problem Two: Withdrawal

Mrs. Carlton had withdrawn from her involvement in her home environment, as described in the nursing history. Her contacts with other patients were limited to one patient, with whom she spent all her time when she was not alone. The withdrawal occurred in the nurse–patient relationship from the beginning when she walked away from the nurse. Her subsequent behavior also showed her reluctance to become involved. She stated that the nurse should work with someone else. She attempted to avoid the nurse by attending a gym class also scheduled at the same time. To deal with this, the nurse was persistent in making contacts with her, even going to the gym and waiting for her. Then the nurse stated directly, "I have chosen to spend this particular time with you which is the only time I have available. I want you to rearrange your schedule to make this hour available." After discussing how to change her schedule, Mrs. Carlton responded to this directive, possibly because she needed so much approval from others to offset her worthless feelings. It resulted in her beginning to spend the allotted time with the nurse, talking about herself, and consequently decreasing her withdrawn, self-involved behavior.

Since relationships were potentially satisfying for Mrs. Carlton, and had been in the past, the nurse encouraged her socialization. At one point the nurse simply said, "I think you would feel better if you would get to know other people here." This suggestion did not seem to make any more impact than others at the time it was stated, but some weeks later Mrs. Carlton said it was one of the most helpful suggestions she had received. To reinforce this suggestion, the nurse also repeatedly asked about Mrs. Carlton's friends, engaged her in conversation with others, and introduced her to others, acting as a role model in some situations. The results from these interventions were especially gratifying to the patient, as social relationships had always been pleasurable to her.

Problem Three: Self-Esteem

Mrs. Carlton's low self-esteem was evident from her comments about herself at home (in the nursing history) and also in the nurse–patient interactions. When the relationship began, she would not talk easily. The nurse found herself talking more, giving suggestions and asking questions. Mrs. Carlton never disagreed with the nurse, but would nod her head in agreement. After a particularly quiet session with Mrs. Carlton, the nurse became frustrated and angry at her apparent lack of interest. This led to the nurse's increasing the questions in such a way that the anger was apparent to Mrs. Carlton. Her response was to say, "I'm not a very good patient, am I?" She felt she had to live up to the nurse's immediate expectations to be worthwhile. The nurse changed her approach to one of decreased questioning, allowing the patient to guide the conversation by bringing up topics important to herself.

Mrs. Carlton did not feel she could perform tasks well enough to undertake them. For example, the nurse asked her to record her feelings between their meetings, using both pictures and the written word. Mrs. Carlton stated she did not "write good." The nurse helped her complete the task the first day and continued to encourage her. She finally agreed to complete the task and did so, after which she continued to apologize for not doing a better job. At this point the nurse said she was pleased that Mrs. Carlton had finished the task, and continued by discussing what she had recorded. Some tasks were not as threatening to her and she was able to accept compliments. This occurred when the nurse saw her embroidery, for example, and also when the nurse complimented her appearance after she had her hair done.

The nurse continued to let Mrs. Carlton know that she was an important and worthwhile person by meeting with her consistently and on time. Mrs. Carlton responded by becoming less self-depreciatory, although she continued to be a very modest person.

Problem Four: Inability to Recognize and Express Feelings

Mrs. Carlton was unable to recognize and express feelings, especially anger. Feelings were especially threatening in relation to those people closest to her— her husband and her son. She reported never getting mad at her husband, and also that she was sexually cold to him. This indicates that love and anger were both difficult for her.

There may have been several reasons for this difficulty, one of them being a fear of losing a loved person. Mrs. Carlton thought that for the child, with his animistic thinking, if anger were expressed toward him, he would retaliate with anger and rejection, thus causing a loss. In addition, if Mrs. Carlton allowed herself to feel very positive about someone, it would increase the hurt she would experience if she were separated from that person. Mrs. Carlton did react strongly to the leaving of two other patients to whom she had become attached. Her comment after the first one had left was this: "I talk to B. (another patient) but I don't want to get too close because I'll feel bad like I did when F. left." The nurse was aware of this problem at a time when a two-week separation was necessary in their relationship. Mrs. Carlton and the nurse had been engaged in some physical exercise designed to bring out angry feelings. Mrs. Carlton did not like these sessions and on this day remained stubbornly quiet about her feelings regarding it. As the nurse prepared to leave for the longer period of time, she sensed Mrs. Carlton's anger. The nurse said, "I hate to leave you feeling the way you are. I'm afraid you'll think I'm not coming back because you were so angry with me." Something about this statement eased the tension. Mrs. Carlton seemed relieved, and goodbyes were said in a more relaxed and spontaneous atmosphere. After the nurse's return two weeks later, Mrs. Carlton was more spontaneous and open than she had ever been before.

The final termination with the nurse was also difficult for Mrs. Carlton, although she was the one leaving, being discharged to go home. At this time, she used the older behavior pattern of being very quiet, not expressing her feelings, even when the nurse encouraged her. The nurse then suggested thoughts and feelings she might be having. At the time the nurse began to walk out the front door, Mrs. Carlton said, "Well, I guess it had to happen sometime."

The other factor involved in Mrs. Carlton's fear of expressing anger was a fear of loss of control. This was especially evident during the sessions using physical activity. This approach was a major one used by the nurse. Activities such as throwing a basketball at a wall and then to each other were used. The sensations from the activity were discussed, which led to feelings and thoughts that were connected with the activity. When throwing the ball directly toward the nurse, Mrs. Carlton said, "You might get hit and your glasses might get broken." The nurse assured Mrs. Carlton of the necessary control by saying, "I don't think that will really happen." Mrs. Carlton found it very hard to behave aggressively when throwing the ball directly toward the nurse, but learned eventually to bounce it quite hard on the floor toward the nurse when she felt angry. The nurse encouraged this physical expression when it occurred. However, up to this time Mrs. Carlton was too threatened to express it so directly, and the nurse used other methods of helping her become aware of and express her feelings.

The nurse attempted to help her become aware of the physical sensations that are a part of emotions. (For example, when one is anxious the heart beats faster.) Mrs. Carlton continually described her feelings as "being nervous." When this happened the nurse asked her to describe it more, how different areas of the body felt, and also what her thoughts were when she was feeling this way. The nurse behaved as a role model in this area also, by describing some of her own feelings and the sensations that accompanied them.

The nurse and the patient also discussed the general subject of anger— how different people handle it, how one can tell that another person is angry, and how one could use some safe outlets for it. Mrs. Carlton's comments about her husband's behavior were interesting. She said that he usually left and did not discuss the difficulty with her; that even though she always knew when he was angry, she could not describe how he looked (facial or body expressions) which would give her indications of his anger. With this kind of behavior from her spouse, one could not plan for her to make great changes in the way she expressed her feelings, unless he also was involved in therapy.

Probably the most profitable approach to this problem was to encourage Mrs. Carlton to express feelings about seemingly trivial matters. This gave her practice in expressing anger without arousing the anxiety over losing someone important to her. For example, in March she had some slight menstrual bleeding and commented that her monthly period had always irritated her and now menopause in general irritated her. The nurse continued a discussion about this and used the session of physical activity to help her express and release the feelings. The nurse said, "As you throw the ball, think about how irritated you are." She was able to be more aggressive in the physical activity during this session.

As time went on, Mrs. Carlton could express more anger about people, as when she was angry at a nurse's aide for not waking up the patients at the normal hour in the morning. Eventually she was more open with her anger toward the nurse. Quite late in the relationship, the nurse was ten minutes late in meeting with Mrs. Carlton. Mrs. Carlton did not greet the nurse with the spontaneous "Hi" that was usual at this stage. As they walked by the nurse's station, Mrs. Carlton looked at the clock and at the nurse's wrist, saying, "Oh, you *do* have a watch." The nurse acknowledged her lateness and asked Mrs. Carlton how she felt about it. At first she rationalized, saying the nurse had to have time to get there from her group at the gym. When pursued about her feelings she admitted she felt a little angry. This was the most direct verbal expression she could give to her anger, and it never extended to the area of the marital relation.

Some changes in the general approach to this problem would have been beneficial. The nurse dealt mainly with anger and did not explore other feelings in depth. However, since Mrs. Carlton had as much trouble with other feelings, a more balanced approach should have been used, with less emphasis on her anger. For example, the guilt that resulted from expressing or even feeling anger would have automatically been decreased by less focus on the anger. (Less guilt would mean increased self-esteem, which Mrs. Carlton, and all depressed persons, badly need.) The nurse needed to also discuss whether the guilt feelings were realistic.

Feelings of closeness, tenderness, and love, and her need for and fear of losing these from others should also have been a major focus for the nurse.

Problem Five: Unrealistic Fears

Mrs. Carlton had unrealistic fears about the future as well as fears about menopause and growing older. These are described in the nursing history. Losses that are eminent during this time of life, and those that are realistic follow: loss of physical abilities, loss of good health, loss of children (as they become independent), loss of loved ones who are older, loss of productivity (of child-bearing capacity), and loss of financial and social standing.

Mrs. Carlton expressed her fears about menopause by telling the nurse about another woman she knew who had hemorrhaged and nearly died. The nurse dealt with this by giving her factual information about menopause.

Her fears about the future centered around finances and the possibilities of physical illness and limitations. To make the future seem a little less grim, the nurse tried to help her discover and maintain interests by suggesting various activities, such as baking, and participating in some with her. The nurse also encouraged her to discuss retirement plans with her husband.

Her fears in general decreased during her hospitalization and she did make some immediate plans for activities when she returned home. However, the success of the discussions in these areas seemed to depend on the decrease of her feelings of worthlessness.

Problem Six: Dependency

Mrs. Carlton was very dependent on other people. Her pattern of dependency is described in the nursing history. When with the nurse, she could not make even very small decisions, could not disagree, and at first could not arrange her schedule to allow time to see the nurse. With encouragement, she did make arrangements with the proper people to have her schedule changed. The decision making came slow. At each session the nurse asked Mrs. Carlton where she would like to go to talk and what she would like to talk about. Usually she said, "I don't know. Where do you want to go to talk?" Then would follow a long silence. When Mrs. Carlton realized that the nurse wanted her to practice making decisions, she began to make an attempt. However, she continually reversed her decision, going back and forth. When Mrs. Carlton was in the process of making decisions, the nurse helped her explore the consequences of the different alternatives she had, and emphasized that a wrong decision might not be as damaging as she imagined.

At times Mrs. Carlton became discouraged with her inability to make decisions, and then the nurse reminded her of the responsibilities and decision making she had assumed before her illness, emphasizing her success with it.

Mrs. Carlton made small advances in this problem area, but it was not realistic to expect great changes, since it was a life pattern for her to use passive, dependent ways of coping.

Problem Seven: Marital Communication

Mrs. Carlton discussed briefly her relationship with her husband. Although she reported no major problems, she did say that they did not discuss things she considered important. When relating what occurred on their weekends together, she reported only conversation about everyday matters. This problem warranted more investigation, and possibly the involvement of the husband with the nurse. However, in the situation in which the nurse was involved, this was impossible due to scheduling, the husband's work hours, and the nurse's limited time.

STUDY GUIDE

The Psychodynamics of Depression

1. What defense mechanisms are used in depression? How do these tie in with the ambivalence, the anger, and the guilt in depression?
2. Describe the obsessive-compulsive personality. What is the purpose of this pre-psychotic way of functioning?
3. Which defense mechanisms are used in the obsessive-compulsive behavior? (Which ones did Mrs. Carlton use?) Give illustrations of how they are used.
4. How does a person like Mrs. Carlton cope with the stresses of life?
5. What are the interpersonal operations in this patient?
6. In what stage of child development does this type of interpersonal relationship occur with the parents?
7. What are the characteristics of this stage?
8. What type of behavior from parents might inhibit normal maturing at this stage, and make the condition ripe for later depression?
9. How does this behavior of the parents affect the child's move toward independence?
10. Why did Mrs. Carlton's defenses break down at the time they did?

The Nursing Care

1. What differences from the usual physical components of depression did you find in this case?
2. How would the care plan differ if these usual physical components of depression would be evident?
3. What would you include in this care plan if this patient had been actively suicidal?
4. What criteria do you use to determine how suicidal a patient is?
5. What is the suicidal potential for this patient?
6. How much dependency should the nurse allow on her/himself from the patient? What factors should the nurse consider in making this decision?

SELECTED READINGS

S. Arieti (ed.), *American Handbook of Psychiatry*, Basic Books, New York, 1959, pp. 345–352, 540–545.

J. Barnett *et al.*, "Involutional Melancholia," *Psychiatric Quarterly*, vol. 27, no. 4, 1953, pp. 654–662.

M. K. Bodie, "When a Patient Threatens Suicide," *Perspectives in Psychiatric Care*, vol. VI, no. 2, 1968, pp. 76–79.

I. M. Burnside, "Grief Work in the Aged Patient," *Nursing Forum*, vol. 8, no. 4, 1969, pp. 416–427.

M. Chapman, "Movement Therapy in the Treatment of Suicidal Patients," *Perspectives in Psychiatric Care*, vol. 9, May–June 1971, pp. 119–122.

L. I. Dublin, *Suicide*, Ronald Press, New York, 1963, pp. 3–45, 153–167.

G. L. Engel, "Grief and Grieving," *American Journal of Nursing*, vol. 64, no. 9, September 1964, pp. 93–98.

O. S. English, "Climacteric Neuroses and Their Management," *Geriatrics*, vol. 9, no. 4, April 1954, pp. 139–145.

N. L. Farberow and E. S. Schneidman (eds.), *The Cry for Help*, McGraw-Hill, New York, 1963, pp. 48–77.

S. Freud, "Mourning and Melancholia," *Collected Papers*, vol. IV, 1934, pp. 152–170. (WM7 F89se V. 4 1925)

F. Fromm-Reichman, *Principles of Intensive Psychotherapy*, The University of Chicago Press, Chicago, 1950, pp. 198–200.

C. K. Hofling and M. M. Leninger, *Basic Psychiatric Concepts in Nursing*, J. B. Lippincott, Philadelphia, 1960, pp. 241–246; 232–237; 279–282; 289–294.

R. A. MacKinnon and R. Michels, *The Psychiatric Interview in Clinical Practice*, W. B. Saunders, Philadelphia, 1971, pp. 174–229.

E. J. McCranie, "Depression, Anxiety, and Hostility," *Psychiatric Quarterly*, vol. 45, no. 1, 1971, pp. 117–133.

M. P. Neylan, "The Depressed Patient," *American Journal of Nursing*, vol. 61, no. 7, July 1961, pp. 77–78.

A. P. Noyes *et al.*, *Psychiatric Nursing*, Macmillan, New York, 1964, pp. 147–153.'

J. Risley, "Nursing Intervention in Depression," *Perspectives in Psychiatric Care*, vol. V, no. 2, 1967, pp. 65–67.

M. S. Schwartz and E. L. Shockley, *The Nurse and the Mental Patient*, John Wiley, New York, 1956, pp. 90–112, 157–198.

F. Shea and E. Hurley, "Hopelessness and Helplessness," *Perspectives in Psychiatric Care*, vol. II, no. 1, 1964, pp. 32–38.

E. S. Shneidman *et al.*, *Clues to Suicide*, McGraw-Hill, New York, 1957, pp. 3–21, 99–118, 153–166, 290–306.

Mrs. Sanders

fifty-five years old

Depression Suicide Attempt/Chronic

Rita Harris Clifford and Margo Lyman Thompson

In the last decade, there has been a major shift in psychiatric care from inpatient settings to outpatient treatment, with the goal of maintaining the individual in his community whenever possible. Mrs. Sanders is a woman who had been marginally adjusted all her life, and when she was fifty-five (in 1969), stressful life situations precipitated an illness of chronic proportions. A nurse in a community mental health center became the individual with major responsibility for her treatment. The care illustrated in this case focuses on a day-to-day reality orientation with a directive approach by the nurse, rather than on the development of insight. The goals of treatment were the relief of symptoms and the production of certain behaviors that would allow Mrs. Sanders to again become a functioning member of her community.

PERSONAL HISTORY

Mrs. Sanders was born in Missouri and was the second of two children. Her father owned and managed several small stores in Missouri while she was in school, and the family moved frequently during that time. Her mother was a housewife and worked part-time in the stores. Mrs. Sanders describes herself as being outgoing as a child and as being active in sports during school. She quit school after the ninth grade because she was "ill." Her father died in 1955 of cancer; her mother died in February 1968 of a myocardial infarction. Her brother now lives in the same town as Mrs. Sanders, and is a very successful businessman.

Mrs. Sanders married a man eight years her senior when she was twenty-two years old. They had no children. She describes their marriage as a happy one, but she states that her husband was not affectionate. He drank beer heavily despite increasing disability due to diabetes. During the last five years of his life, she often accompanied him to taverns, which caused her many guilt feelings because of her strong religious beliefs. Mrs. Sanders's mother had lived with Mr. and Mrs. Sanders for ten years before Mr. Sanders's death in 1967.

For many years, Mrs. Sanders had sought medical treatment for numerous physical problems. These problems were diagnosed as chronic thrombophlebitis, pulmonary embolism, psychophysiological cardiovascular reaction, obesity, hypertension, and migraine headaches. She had many surgical procedures, including appendectomy, removal of abdominal abscess, partial and total hysterectomies, and cholecystectomy.

Mrs. Sanders first experienced depression in December of 1967, when her husband died of diabetic complications. In February 1968, her mother died while trying to revive Mrs. Sanders, who had fainted. The depressive symptoms re-occurred. She improved somewhat during that summer, but again began having symptoms six weeks prior to being seen by a physician in the psychiatry outpatient department in November 1968. She sought psychiatric treatment because of anorexia, insomnia, protracted crying spells, and numerous somatic complaints (headaches, fainting, and angina).

During the course of treatment in the psychiatric outpatient department, Mrs. Sanders focused on the symptomatology of her depression. She talked at length about her sleeplessness and her lack of appetite. She cried easily and frequently and had many physical complaints such as dizziness, fainting, muscular aches and pains, headaches, heart pounding, pains in her chest, and constipation. She frequently spoke about her mother and expressed guilt for her mother's death. In addition, she constantly made self-depreciatory comments such as, "I never could keep my house as clean as my mother could." "I never was very smart." "I'm so ugly, I don't know how anyone could like me." She expressed hostility toward her brother and her mother-in-law because she felt they did not like her and did not treat her kindly. At this time, she was placed on Librium 25 mg four times daily. This had little effect on her symptoms, so she was placed on Mellaril 100 mg four times daily, which resulted in some decrease in her anxiety level.

COURSE OF TREATMENT

On February 3, 1969, Mrs. Sanders was referred to a mental health center, where she was evaluated. She was assigned to be seen regularly by a nurse in the outpatient clinic for medication supervision and supportive psychotherapy. In reviewing the course of previous psychiatric treatment, the nurse found that efforts directed exclusively toward the development of insight were unproductive. She decided to allow the verbalization of some feelings attached to past events. Talking about present events, feelings and behavior was encouraged and rewarded, with the focus being on Mrs. Sanders's behavior and how they could be modified. During these first sessions, Mrs. Sanders continued to talk about her symptoms and her feelings about her mother, husband, and brother. She verbalized only very positive feelings about her mother and husband. She could give no examples of faults of theirs except for those for which she took the responsibility; for example, husband's drinking, her mother's expectation of perfection from Mrs. Sanders, and discord between her mother and her husband.

She had done office work prior to her husband's death, but since the onset of her depression, she has been living on social security benefits from her husband and disability benefits for herself. She and her brother own the house in which she lives. The brother refuses to pay any of the taxes or upkeep on the house, which angers Mrs. Sanders.

Mrs. Sanders verbalized feelings of extreme loneliness. She felt unloved and useless. She would often spend all day in bed, then could not sleep at night. She stated that she had no energy to do her housework, shopping, or anything. Her only form of socialization was her church work, but during her extremely low periods, she refused to attend church. She stated that her only friend was the pastor of the church.

Despite her anorexia, Mrs. Sanders was quite obese (height, 5 feet, 1 inch; weight, 81 kg). When she first began coming to the mental health center, her appearance was quite unkempt. Her hair was usually dirty and uncombed; she wore either no makeup or only bright red lipstick, carelessly applied; her clothes were ill-fitting, unpressed, and unattractive. As treatment continued, her appearance was usually a highly reliable indication of her emotional state. When she said she felt better, she looked cleaner, neater, more attractive; when she felt worse, she looked as described above.

During her course of treatment, Mrs. Sanders was on varying doses of Librium, Valium, and Tofranil. On the second anniversary of her mother's death (February 15, 1970), she was seen at the mental health center by the nurse. At that time, Mrs. Sanders was extremely depressed. She appeared extremely disheveled and was exhibiting behaviors that had not been seen in some time; that is, crying and tremulousness. She reported having difficulty sleeping and a marked decrease in appetite. She spent the entire session making self-depreciatory remarks and hopeless statements, but denied suicidal thoughts. Nonetheless, the nurse was concerned about the possibility of suicide. Mrs. Sanders was given an appointment for the following week and instructions to call either the mental health center or suicide prevention center if she should feel worse or contemplate suicide. The dosage of Tofranil was increased to 25 mg three times daily and Valium was continued at 5 mg twice daily.

On February 19, she called the nurse stating she was afraid she was "getting sicker." The nurse made a home visit, during which she determined that Mrs. Sanders was in need of hospitalization. She arranged for her admission to the state hospital, where Mrs. Sanders remained until March 3. She was discharged much improved, and follow-up treatment continued at the mental health center.

The nurse felt that she was maintaining the improvement noted at the time of her discharge from the state hospital. However, on April 16, 1970, her pastor called the nurse stating he had just found Mrs. Sanders in a semicomatose state. Mrs. Sanders had told him she had taken an overdose of sleeping pills. The nurse recommended that he bring Mrs. Sanders to the emergency room. Upon her arrival there, she was admitted to the medical intensive care unit. On the seventh day of hospitalization, she was dismissed with diagnosis of "exogenous obesity" and "depressive reaction" and was referred to the mental health center for continued treatment.

Dramatic improvement in the depressive symptoms was noted by the nurse when treatment resumed. Many of the same concerns which had been important since the beginning of treatment remained unresolved. However, the ways in which Mrs. Sanders dealt with daily living situations seemed to have changed. She was able to participate actively in her church once more and had an observable increase in energy level. Mrs. Sanders began to assert herself in her relations without being obsessed afterward about her actions. During this time, the nurse's approach became less directive and more supportive. The need for care still existed, and Mrs. Sanders continued to be seen at the center, but less frequently.

NURSING INTERVENTION

The following outline is an excerpt from the care plan written by the nurse and is illustrative of the primary areas of concern identified and some of the nursing actions undertaken.

IDENTIFIED AREAS OF CONCERN	NURSING ACTIVITIES

1. Past medical history
   a. Chronic thrombophlebitis—pulmonary embolism with hemoptesis
   b. Psychophysiological cardiovascular reaction
   c. Chronic obesity
   d. Chronic hypertension
   e. Migraine headache
	Observation
	Checked routinely with the physician under whose care Mrs. Sanders remained for her medical problems.

2. Depression
   a. Dynamics of depression
      (1) Loss of love object
	Encouraged talk about loss of husband and mother.

IDENTIFIED AREAS OF CONCERN (*continued*)	NURSING ACTIVITIES (*continued*)
(2) Ambivalence toward love object	Evaluated her relationships with them. She had them idealized—attempted to help her see them more realistically. Many of her statements showed hidden hostility toward her husband and her mother, but she could not openly admit this. Pointed these feelings out to her, at the same time reassuring her that many of them were reasonable and acceptable.
(3) Guilt about ambivalence	Pointed out that ambivalence was acceptable and normal in a relationship. One can never completely love someone.
(4) Introjection of hostility	Listened to obsession with causing mother's death. Tried to gently lead her to realization that she did not cause it consciously. No attempt to deal with possible unconscious wish for mother's death. Finally told her positively that she had not caused her mother's death . . . that she appeared to enjoy beating herself over the head with this . . . that I didn't feel this was helping her and I didn't want to hear about it anymore. She appeared to accept this strong statement and subsequently reported that she did not think about it constantly as she had before.
b. Isolation (1) Feeling useless (2) Feeling lack of interest in self and environment (3) Feeling unwanted and unloved	Together we made out a daily schedule for her to follow, listing all activities during the day. She checked the activities off as she did them and brought the list back to me. Suggested that she return to church and become active in circle, which she did. Encouraged socialization with a club and bowling teams. She attempted these with much verbal pushing from me at first. Told her to take a babysitting job (which was offered to her), which she did. Dealt with relationship with brother—pointed out to her that it was unlikely that the relationship would ever change.

IDENTIFIED AREAS OF CONCERN (*continued*)	NURSING ACTIVITIES (*continued*)
	She would have to live with it and not spend time being obsessed with it. After talking about it with her a number of times, I began stopping her when she brought it up and helped her look at ways of handling the problems without his help.
	Indicated with both words and actions that I considered her important, that I was concerned about her, that our relationship was meaningful to me.
c. Somatic complaints 　(1)　Muscular aches 　(2)　Nausea 　(3)　Tremors 　(4)　Back pain 　(5)　Weakness	Refused to talk about them. Diverted attention with goal of extinguishing complaints.
	Encouraged activity and socialization as above.
	Was alert to any actual physical problems or change in types or intensity of usual complaints.
d. Physical components 　(1)　Insomnia	Talked about excessive coffee intake, suggested caffeine-free coffee.
	Encouraged re-establishing of old, more successful, sleeping habits.
	Suggested diversional activities before bed; for example, bath, reading, listening to radio, if these helped to relax.
	Arranged time schedule of regular daily medications so that the optimum relaxation took place at bedtime.
(2)　Anorexia	Suggested small meals, balanced diet, watching fattening foods (keep in mind obesity, but don't want to lose too much too fast). Reinforced necessity for eating.
(3)　Crying	Used directive approach: "Stop crying." "When you start, do something else—wash dishes, clothes."
(4)　Appearance	Said, "You look depressed." Encouraged, using washing hair, ironing clothes as activities.

IDENTIFIED AREAS OF CONCERN (*continued*)	NURSING ACTIVITIES (*continued*)
	Complimented when she looked nice, but was matter-of-fact. Observed for action and side effects of medications: Librium, Tofranil, Valium.
(5) Motor retardation	Directed her activities: worked out a daily time schedule; encouraged activities of a gross motor nature.
e. Suicidal feelings	Was alert for abrupt change in intensity of symptoms, hopeless and self-depreciatory talk. Pointed out to Mrs. Sanders this abrupt change when it occurred. Verbalized concern about suicidal possibility to Mrs. Sanders. Accepted her denial of this possibility as necessary for her, but maintained own conviction that this was a possibility. Gave her specific instructions about who to contact should suicidal feelings occur. Made an immediate home visit after her call to objectively evaluate situation.

STUDY GUIDE

1. Can the grieving process be related to Mrs. Sanders's situation? How?
2. How does the nurse identify which patients could benefit from the directive, reality-oriented approach described in the case? List the pros and cons of such an approach.
3. What are other areas of concern which should have been identified by the nurse?
4. What other nursing activities may have been appropriate and helpful?
5. How did the nurse identify a suicidal potential in Mrs. Sanders on February 15?
6. What is the significance of the date February 15 to Mrs. Sanders?
7. What reasons could the nurse have had for not hospitalizing Mrs. Sanders at that time?
8. How can one explain a suicide attempt soon after being released from the hospital "much improved?"

9. What might the nurse have done to prevent the suicide attempt after hospitalization?
10. Discuss the possible reasons for the long-lasting improvement after the suicide attempt.
11. Were Mrs. Sanders's pre-depression coping mechanisms related to her symptoms in depression? If so, how?
12. Discuss the feelings you, as a nurse, might have should a patient with whom you have been working attempt or commit suicide.

SELECTED READINGS

E. Ansel and R. McGee, "Attitudes Toward Suicide Attempters," *Bulletin of Suicidology*, National Clearinghouse for Mental Health Information, no. 8, Fall 1971.

K. Bell, "The Nurse's Role in Suicide Prevention," *Bulletin of Suicidology*, National Clearinghouse for Mental Health Information, no. 6, Spring 1970.

F. Crumb, "Limited Social Recovery: Further Discussion of a Depressive Behavior Pattern," *Perspectives in Psychiatric Care*, vol. IV, no. 3, 1966, pp. 26–30.

F. Cutter, "Suicide: The Wish, The Act, The Outcome," *Life Threatening Behavior*, vol. 1, no. 2, Summer 1971.

F. Evans, *Psychosocial Nursing*, Macmillan, New York, 1971, chaps. 1, 2, 6, 7, and 9.

C. K. Holfling *et al.*, *Basic Psychiatric Concepts in Nursing*, J. B. Lippincott, Philadelphia, 1967, pp. 285–312.

E. Jacobson, *Depression*, International Universities Press, New York, 1971, chaps. 1, 3, 4, and 6.

J. Risley, "Nursing Intervention in Depression," *Perspectives in Psychiatric Care*, vol. V, no. 2, 1967, pp. 65–67.

M. Schwartz and E. Shockley, *The Nurse and the Mental Patient*, Russell Sage Foundation, New York, Revised 1965, pp. 167–181.

Mr. Carpenter
fifty-five years old

Myocardial Infarction*/ Acute
Jean A. Yokes

GENERAL DESCRIPTION

Mr. Carpenter is a fifty-five-year-old widower who lives in a small trailer camp in Kansas City, Kansas. He is 5 feet, 6 inches tall, and weighs 84 kg. A ruddy facial complexion is crowned beyond a receding hairline by thick, wavy hair, once black and now predominantly gray. He has a warm, appealing smile, and his face becomes flushed when he laughs. His voice is confident, hardy, and forthright.

HISTORY OF PRESENT ILLNESS

On Labor Day, 1970, there had been a family reunion in which Mr. Carpenter had participated in water skiing and several baseball games. The following evening, September 8, while reclining on the sofa in his trailer, he began having substernal, dull, aching chest pain. Thinking at first that his stomach was the cause of the distress, he took an antacid. He had read about the signs of a heart attack and it occurred to him that this might be the cause of his pain, but he was inclined to deny it.

When the antacids failed to give him relief, he and his son walked around the trailer court several hours in an attempt to relieve the pain. Five hours after the onset of the chest pain, Mr. Carpenter became more concerned as the intensity of the pain increased and the pain began radiating across his chest and down his left arm. He then asked his son to take him to the Kansas University Medical Center, where he was admitted to the intensive care unit with a diagnosis of an acute anterior wall myocardial infarction.

---

* The nursing observations and intervention were provided by Mrs. Shirley Sleeker, R.N., M.S.N., a graduate student in nursing in 1970 at the time this case was compiled.

HISTORY OF PAST-HEALTH STATUS

Mr. Carpenter recalled only two previous episodes of illness. The first was an "upset stomach" in 1952, which was diagnosed at Mayo Clinic as an ulcer. A bland diet and Probanthine was prescribed. Mr. Carpenter said that he resigned himself to following the diet. He admitted to deviating from it occasionally, but basically his diet habits changed to avoid abdominal distress. This change in dietary habit would seem to indicate strong self-discipline.

The second illness was in 1958, when he was hospitalized for two days following an allergic reaction to tetanus toxoid, which he had received after a laceration and fracture of his left hand. Mr. Carpenter described the hospitalization as "confining," saying he wanted "to be on my own again." This reaction indicates an independent nature.

SOCIAL HISTORY

Two weeks after his family came to the United States, Mr. Carpenter was born. His mother, father, three sisters, and four brothers settled in New York City, where his father did heavy labor. After Mr. Carpenter's father began an asphalt business, the family migrated between Florida and New York, depending on the seasonal changes affecting that business.

Mr. Carpenter began his own family at eighteen. After his wife's sudden death at twenty-eight, he raised their twin daughters and son with the help of his mother. Now adults, his children have families of their own. Mr. Carpenter has a total of fifteen grandchildren. Although each of the three families and Mr. Carpenter live in separate trailers, they always move together. Mr. Carpenter appeared to be the dominant member of the families.

Mr. Carpenter's education extended to the ninth grade. He said he read a good deal in his leisure time and also learned much from his travels. His main interests in life, however, centered around physical activities, especially sports. For example, he had actively participated in football, baseball, and water skiing, and, because he enjoyed nature and the out-of-doors, he hunted and fished several times a year.

ECONOMIC HISTORY

Mr. Carpenter had done either heavy labor or asphalt work most of his life. At the time of his heart attack, he owned and managed an asphalt business which was located in Kansas City or Texas, depending on seasonal conditions. He described this business as a family business, with his son and two sons-in-law doing most of the work involving heavy machinery, while he planned and organized the jobs. This work having been profitable, Mr. Carpenter never was without the basic comforts.

DAILY HABITS

Mr. Carpenter usually began his day at 6 A.M. and retired at 10:30 P.M. His work hours varied according to the weather and job requirements, but he often worked until dusk. If not working late, he usually became involved in some physical sport.

Self-sufficient, with no particular food dislikes, Mr. Carpenter prepared his own meals, usually of beef, potatoes, and vegetables. He usually showered in the evening.

MEDICAL REGIME

The physician's orders were bedrest with bedside commode, morphine sulfate for pain, Colace 100 mg P.O. at h.s., Maalox 30 cc, p.r.n., vital signs, continuous EKG monitoring, oxygen at 5 liters per minute, intravenous lidocaine drip, 1 mg/ml in 1000 cc 5% dextrose/water and 1,500 calorie, low sodium, bland ulcer diet.

NURSING ASSESSMENT

The initial nursing assessment of Mr. Carpenter was made in relation to cardiopulmonary status, fluid and electrolyte status, status of basic needs, and mental health status.

Assessment of the *cardiopulmonary status* determined normal color of mucous membranes and skin of the extremities. The skin was warm to the touch. Mr. Carpenter complained of two episodes of chest pain on the first hospitalized day. The apical pulse was 64–70 and regular at time of assessment. The radial pulse was strong without pulse deficit. (Three to four premature ventricular contractions per minute had been noted on the cardiac monitor oscilloscope until treatment with lidocaine had been initiated.) The blood pressure was 112/70 to 120/78. Pulmonary rales or a third heart sound were not heard upon auscultation.

Assessment of *fluid and electrolyte status* revealed intact skin with good turgor. Mr. Carpenter's muscular tone was excellent. He did not complain of feeling weak, and his sensorium was clear as determined by orientation to time, place, and recent events. Mr. Carpenter had control of bladder and bowels. He experienced two episodes of diaphoresis during the first hospitalized night. His appetite was good and his lower denture and remaining good teeth permitted proper mastication of food.

Because of activity restriction imposed by medical orders, Mr. Carpenter was not able to meet *basic hygienic* needs such as bathing himself. He was, however, allowed to feed himself without apparent compromise to his cardiopulmonary system.

An evaluation of Mr. Carpenter's *mental health status* indicated some depression but use of positive coping-adaptation mechanisms. Frequent visits by many friends and family members were not limited because of his stable physical status. These visitors provided positive support, affection, diversion, and motivation to help him through his adjustment to living with heart disease. Family members later exhibited interest in Mr. Carpenter's future welfare by attending dietary classes.

Some business advice was given to a son. Control of business matters from the bedside also provided positive factors for short- and long-term rehabilitation.

Mr. Carpenter related humorous experiences, possibly using humor to relieve the anxiety he experienced as a result of the heart attack. He related he was unsure what the heart attack meant to him and his future. A tight facial expression with wrinkled eyebrows was noted. His eyes intently followed the nurse during the simplistic explanation of the heart, how it works as a pump, and what occurred to the heart at the time of a heart attack or coronary occlusion. Mr. Carpenter questioned how cholesterol affected the heart and the role of diet to prevent future heart attacks. This concern over diet and activity seemed to reflect a positive attitude toward following preventive health practices. Past health habits discussed in the history also reflected positive preventive health practices. Mr. Carpenter was aware of and spoke frequently of the other patients in the room and their discomforts. This concern for events outside himself would indicate that his degree of depression due to illness and hospitalization was mild. In summary, Mr. Carpenter exhibited strong mental health factors which would be utilized to attain maximum long-term rehabilitation and return to work.

COURSE OF HOSPITALIZATION

Mr. Carpenter spent the *first week* of hospitalization in the medical intensive care unit for constant nursing observation of his physical status. His physical status was uncomplicated. His serum enzyme elevations were CPK:548 mg, SGOT:160 mg, and LDH:2,144 mg.

Those individuals who suffer an acute anterior myocardial infarction are prone to develop heart block that may require insertion of a transvenous pacemaker. The individual with an uncomplicated first myocardial infarction has an excellent prognosis and can hope for resumption of most of his former activities. Those individuals who have had sedentary life styles before first infarction can, through a gradated exercise regime during rehabilitation, gain a greater exercise tolerance and hopefully improve coronary circulation and cardiopulmonary status.

Mr. Carpenter spent the *second week* of hospitalization on a general medical unit. Chest pain was absent. He expressed anxiety about leaving the intensive care unit, though he realized discharge from the unit was an indication of improved physical status. He had some disturbance in sleep as evidenced by insomnia. The dreams he had were a way of relieving the anxieties created by the heart attack and subsequent hospitalization. His physical activity was increased. A Class IV hyperlipoproteinemia diet was prescribed.

Discharge from the hospital occurred during the *third week* following the acute myocardial infarction. Mr. Carpenter expressed concern about the physical activity he was allowed. He was impatient to return to his former life style and wanted to know what restrictions would be imposed.

POST-HOSPITALIZATION COURSE

Three home visits were made by the nurse. At the conclusion of the third visit, both Mr. Carpenter and the nurse felt no need for future visits. Mr. Carpenter could call the nurse if particular concerns occurred. If chest pain recurred and was not relieved by rest and nitroglycerine, Mr. Carpenter would return to the hospital. This unrelieved chest pain might indicate an extension of his previous infarction or a second infarction.

During the home visits the nurse elicited Mr. Carpenter's concerns which were alleviated by providing information, i.e., clarification of diet regime, the role gradual weight loss played in reducing the work load of the heart, gradual increase in exercise such as walking, and gradual return to a full day's work. Mr. Carpenter was taught stress level indicators such as increase in pulse rate over 110 and presence of fatigue. He later discussed his increasing ability to control tension when his sons expressed opposite viewpoints on business matters. Mr. Carpenter was also learning to relinquish full managerial responsibilities, and self-confidence was returning along with his increase in physical activity. Ever present was his hope that his health practices would prevent a second heart attack.

SUMMARY

The nursing process involved (1) collection of data pertinent to Mr. Carpenter's illness: the precipitating events, previous and present coping-adaptation behavior, and hospitalization events; (2) utilization of data to plan and provide nursing intervention; and (3) evaluation of nursing intervention.

STUDY GUIDE

1. What is the clinical picture of a person who is experiencing an acute myocardial infarction? What are the immediate nursing interventions?
2. What laboratory data are needed to help substantiate the diagnosis of acute myocardial infarction?

3. What changes occur on a 12 lead electrocardiogram that indicate ischemia and injury to the myocardium?
4. What are the normal serum enzyme levels of SGOT, CPK, and LDH? What do abnormal findings suggest in this case?
5. Since electrical instability of the heart is the leading sequela following an acute myocardial infarction, detection of warning arrhythmias is important. What corrective nursing actions may be taken (as hospital policy dictates) to prevent the occurrence of life-threatening arrhythmias?
6. What aggressive actions are taken when lethal arrhythmias occur?
7. In an individual not being monitored, how would one recognize and distinguish between asystole and ventricular fibrillation? Discuss the definitive measures for each.
8. In most individuals, what major coronary artery would be involved in an acute inferior (diaphragmatic) infarct? In an acute anteriorseptal infarct? What normal pathways of the electrical conduction system nourished by these arteries would be involved in each area of infarction?
9. What is the aggressive surgical management for coronary occlusive disease?
10. What electrical safety factors should be maintained in the patient's environment?
11. What should the patient and family be taught about the temporary and permanent pacemaker?
12. Discuss the mechanisms of congestive heart failure and cardiogenic shock, their early warning signs and symptoms, and the medical/nursing management.
13. What are thought to be the personality characteristics of the "coronary prone" individual?
14. What emotional reactions can the nurse expect of the patient with a myocardial infarct? Of the patient's family? What nursing interventions may be anticipated to alleviate these reactions?
15. What nursing intervention can the nurse provide the patient and family to alleviate anxiety and fear when the patient is transferred from the CCU/ICU to the intermediate or general medical unit?
16. What are the rehabilitation considerations and the nursing intervention?
17. Discuss diet in relation to the five types of hyperlipoproteinemias.

SELECTED READINGS

K. G. Andreoli *et al., Comprehensive Cardiac Care,* 2d ed., C. V. Mosby, St. Louis, 1971.

E. R. Brener, "Surgery for Coronary Artery Disease," *AJN,* March 1972, pp. 469–473.

G. D. Carnes, "Understanding the Cardiac Patient's Behavior," *AJN*, June 1971, pp. 1187–1188.

N. H. Cassem *et al.*, "Reactions of Coronary Patients to the CCU Nurse," *AJN*, February 1970, pp. 319–325.

E. L. Coodley, "Significance of Serum Enzymes," *AJN*, February 1968, pp. 301–304.

D. Dubin, *Rapid Interpretation of EKG's*, Cover Publishing, Tampa, Florida, 1970.

S. Foster and K. G. Andreoli, "Behavior Following Acute Myocardial Infarction," *AJN*, November 1970, pp. 2344–2348.

L. E. Graham, "Patients' Perceptions in the CCU," *AJN*, September 1969, pp. 1921–1922.

G. L. Griffith, "Sexuality and the Cardiac Patient," *Heart and Lung*, January–February 1973, pp. 70–73.

A. Hahn and N. Dolan, "After Coronary Care Then What?" *AJN*, November 1970, pp. 2350–2352.

R. Merkel and C. M. Brown, "Evaluating Feeding Activities in a CCU," *AJN*, November 1970, pp. 2348–2350.

La V. Sharp and B. Rabin, *Nursing in the Coronary Care Unit*, J. B. Lippincott, Philadelphia, 1970.

D. E. Sobel, "Personalization on the CCU," *AJN*, July 1969, pp. 1439–1442.

J. A. Yokes, "The Family of a Myocardial Infarction Patient," (ed.) Hymovitch and Barnard, *Readings: Family Nursing*, McGraw-Hill, New York, 1973 (to be published).

Special Supplement: "The Patient with a Myocardial Infarction," *AJN*, November 1964, C-1-32.

Mr. Prince
fifty-seven years old

Aortic Valve Replacement for Aortic Stenosis/Acute

Lily Larson

Mr. Marvin Prince, fifty-seven-year-old Caucasian, works in a downtown high-rise apartment building in a metropolitan area as a head night janitor. He lives with his fifty-four-year-old wife and fourteen-year-old adopted son, Rob, in the apartment building. He is a volunteer fireman and has enjoyed working with Boy Scouts for several years. He is proud of his work record as a janitor, missing very few work days over a period of fifteen to twenty years until December 1971. Mr. Prince attempted to obtain better paying jobs, but he said he lacked the required education and training. He is a high school graduate.

Although it was known that he had a heart murmur, he served several years in World War II. During this time, he had a tonsillectomy and removal of impacted wisdom teeth, complicated by osteomyelitis of the jaw. He also had a bilateral inguinal herniorrhaphy. He cannot remember having had rheumatic fever. During Miss Lee's first visit with Mr. Prince on June 23, 1972, his day of admission, he volunteered that he was thankful for all his friends who, when they learned he was to have heart surgery, donated more blood to the blood bank than was needed for his surgery.

Mr. Prince had smoked about two packs of cigarettes for the past thirty-four years. He stopped smoking in March 1972. Since then, his coughing and expectoration decreased greatly. Symptoms which led him to consult his physician in February 1972 were leg swelling, dyspnea upon walking stairs, and orthopnea. He was hospitalized in February 1972 for eleven days, at which time he was taking diuretics and digitalis. His weight dropped from 102.7 kg to 90 kg. He said his normal weight of 79.5 kg is about right for his height of 5 feet, 7 inches, moderate build.

Mr. Prince has one brother, age fifty-five, with "heart trouble"; and a sister, age fifty-two, with severe emphysema. He said he was afraid he would "end up" having emphysema, and with encouragement from his wife and his physician, he decided to throw his cigarettes away.

Dr. Howard, Mr. Prince's physician, referred him to the cardiology department for an evaluation on April 10, 1972. At this time, he was taking Lanoxin 0.5 mg four times daily, Hygrotin (Chlorthaledone) 5 mg three times a week, and a 1,500-mg salt-restricted diet.

Mr. Prince was admitted to the hospital on April 10, 1972, for cardiac catheterization. The physical examination at this time showed blood pressure 140/85; pulse 80, irregular; respiration 18; temperature 37°C. Jugular venous distention to 10 cm. Chest: increased anteroposterior diameter, decreased respiratory exchange. Breath sounds distant. There was a grade III/IV systolic ejection murmur in the second right intercostal space radiating to the carotid. There was also a grade II/VI holosystolic murmur at the apex which was transmitted to the lower left sternal border of the left axilla. Examination of the abdomen revealed that the liver was displaced 1 to 2 cm below the right costal margin. Peripheral distal pulses were good.

Laboratory tests and x ray. The following laboratory tests were normal: complete blood count, fasting blood sugar, blood urea nitrogen, sodium, potassium, chlorides, carbon dioxide, calcium and phosphorus and liver function tests. The following tests were abnormal: cholesterol 276 mg %, and triglycerides 110 mg %. Electrocardiogram revealed atrial fibrillation. There was also left ventricular hypertrophy with secondary ST and T wave changes. There was a suggestion of an apical or inferior myocardial infarction of old age. Chest x ray was consistent with aortic valve disease.

CARDIAC CATHETERIZATION REPORT

Somewhat low cardiac output of 4.4 liters/min; cardiac index 2.2 liters/min/M2; normal right atrial pressure at 3 mean; P.A. pressure of 32/18; L.A. pressure normal with a mean of 7. Left ventricular and diastolic pressure was 195/0–10, compared to simultaneous peripheral pressure of 125/70. The peak systolic gradient was 70 mm Hg and the mean gradient was 35 mm Hg, giving a calculated valve area of 0.67 cm x2. The normal atrial pressure is against severe mitral insufficiency but symptomatic primarily as a result of significant aortic stenosis.

Mr. Prince was discharged the day after his cardiac catheterization. His medical diagnosis was

1. Inactive rheumatic heart disease
2. Aortic stenosis
3. Congestive heart failure
4. Atrial fibrillation

Mr. Prince entered University Hospital on June 23, 1972, for cardiac surgery.

His physical examination on June 23, 1972 (excluding his heart problem and its complications) was essentially negative, except for slight dysarthria of his fingers, slight narrowing of the arterioles of his retina, and slight enlargement of the prostate.

Heart findings: Auscultation—sounds decreased at base. Systolic murmur heard best at the apex and radiates toward the left axilla. Murmur also heard at second intercostal space and right sternal border. Murmur heard throughout systole—high-pitched. No friction rub. Lower extremity pulses are palpable but less than normal.

His admission weight was 87.7 kg, a loss of 2.5 kg, since February.

Medical orders on June 23 were

1. 1,500 mg salt liquid diet
2. Prepare for surgery for June 25
3. Lab: C.B.C., U.A., pro time, clotting and bleeding, BUN, SGOT, FBS, CI, K, CO_2 Ca, PO_4, albumin.
4. Chest x ray

Results of the above tests: hemoglobin 17.8; hematocrit 52; white blood count 10,400, segmented 66, lymphocytes 22, monocytes 9, eosinophiles 3; platelets 258,000, urea IV. 16; creatinine 1.0, sodium 139, potassium 3, chlorides 100; carbon dioxide 30, calcium 4.8, phosphorus 1.8. Total protein 7.4, albumin 4.4, globulin 3.0. Prothrombin time: 13.4 (control) 13.5 patient, bleeding 2½ minutes, coagulation 13 minutes. Fasting blood sugar normal. Liver function tests: bilirubin 0.6 total; alkaline phosphatase 3.2, SGOT 15; urinalysis negative; chest film negative.

On the day of admission, the nurse, Miss Lee, showed Mr. Prince the surgical intensive care unit and told him he would be there several days following surgery because he could be watched more closely and that all "heart" patients who have surgery come to the surgical intensive care unit for close watching.

Miss Lee visited Mr. Prince in the late afternoon to assess Mr. Prince's need during the preoperative period. Mr. Prince seemed to have a good understanding of the purpose and desired outcome of his surgery, which was to be removal of the stenosed aortic valve and replacement with a prosthetic valve. His response to his visit to the intensive care unit was, "I hope they won't have to use all that machinery on me." Miss Lee explained to him why and how oxygen may be used, the purpose of the chest tubes, urinometer, frequent vital sign checks, the cardiac monitor, intravenous infusions, and intermittent positive pressure breathing. He appeared attentive and said he was glad they had a place where personnel and equipment are available at all times.

Mr. Prince shared a room with Mr. Johnson, a fifty-eight-year-old blind man who was to go home in a few days following open heart surgery. Mr. Johnson probably was Mr. Prince's best teacher and supporter before surgery.

Mr. Johnson demonstrated to Mr. Prince, at the request of Miss Lee, how to deep breathe and cough. Mr. Johnson seemed eager to help. He proceeded as follows while Mr. Prince was asked to follow his directions:

"Place your hands on your ribs so you can feel your chest move. It's easier if you sit up straight. Relax your abdominal muscles. Breathe in as much air as you can while you expand your chest. Tighten your abdominal muscles while you purse your lips and expel all the air. Then breathe in again and cough as you expel the deep breath. It's easy to do now, but hurts like hell after your operation unless you really support your chest. You'll have a lot of 'stuff to get up.' The breathing machine (IPPB) helps you cough up what's in your lungs."

Miss Lee informed Mr. Johnson that Mr. Prince was following directions very well. Mr. Johnson said

"Right after surgery, I gave a few hacks with my throat so the nurses up there jammed a tube down my throat and I had to cough. That really hurt a lot, so that taught me a lesson to do some deep down coughing. It's better to practice before."

Mr. Prince said he had been stuck by needles quite a lot and wondered why. Miss Lee, who was aware of the kinds of tests being ordered, explained that the findings of these tests would help the physician determine the kinds of fluids and medicine and/or form of treatment. Miss Lee told him he would have several tests done and have several chest x rays to determine the status of the cardiovascular system and that very likely blood tests would be taken quite frequently in the intensive care unit. Because Mr. Prince appeared attentive to Mr. Johnson and seemed curious to know more, Miss Lee felt that Mr. Prince was more curious to know about reasons for intravenous therapy oxygen, monitoring, etc. He told Miss Lee that he had read a lot about heart transplants and wondered how different a valve prosthesis might be as compared with a new heart.

Some information valuable for nursing care that Mr. Prince offered in the interview was that he had trouble sleeping at night perhaps because he usually slept during the day. His usual pattern was to sleep from 6 A.M. until 1 P.M. with a nap early in the evening.

JUNE 24

Reported on nurse's notes: Slept well after midnight. Weight 85.7 kg.
    Medical orders:

Procaine penicillin, 6 M units I.M. 9–1–5–9–1–5
Streptomycin 500 mg I.M. 9–9
Prostaphylin 1 g P.O. 9–1–5–9–1–5

IPPB q. 4 h. from 8 A.M.–10 P.M.

Chloral hydrate 500 mg P.O. h.s.

1,500 mg salt-restricted liquid diet

May have water until 8 A.M.

Cross match 6 units of blood

Hexacloraphene soap bath t.i.d., routine shave

D.C. Lanoxin and Hygrotin

During the afternoon, Miss Lee visited Mr. Prince to answer questions Mr. Prince and his family might have and to assess his readiness for surgery. Mr. Prince said that he was anxious to have the surgery completed, and fur- thermore said he did not know that the outcome of his recovery depended so much on what he did regarding exercises, breathing, and coughing. He said that this had not been emphasized when he had had his other operations. Mr. Prince practiced the range of motion exercises that had been demon- strated by the nurse. He performed these completely and with ease and knew why they were beneficial. Mrs. Prince and Rob observed during this practice period and said they would expect him to perform again that evening. Miss Lee checked Mr. Prince's pedal pulses, which were easily palpable. His apical pulse was (irregular) 100. Blood pressure was 160/90.

Mr. Prince talked at length about his friends who had contributed blood and that he hoped he would be able to thank each one of them. Mrs. Prince told him that she had telephoned several of them. As if to reassure himself, he said, "The resident said I'm in good shape for the operation." Both Mrs. Prince and Rob tried to appear calm and spoke to Mr. Prince about happenings at home. Miss Lee answered some questions Mrs. Prince and Rob had about time of surgery and what they might be doing while waiting.

JUNE 25—DAY OF SURGERY

Mr. Prince slept well with the aid of chloral hydrate at bedtime.

8:00 A.M.: Foley catheter to direct closed drainage by medical student.

11:00 A.M.: Innover 2.5 mg and Scopolomine 0.5 mg. I.M. given by nurse.

Mrs. Prince and Rob visited a short time in the morning.

11:30 A.M.: Mr. Prince was assisted to the operating room cart by the nurse and the operating room orderly. Mrs. Prince and Rob went to the waiting room, informing the nurse where they were going for lunch. The nurse informed Mrs. Prince that she would be notified when Mr. Prince's surgery was com pleted and when he would return to the intensive care unit and where she could speak with the physician.

Report of operation: Diagnosis—Aortic stenosis and insufficiency calcified aortic valve. Operation—Replacement of aortic valve (Starr-Edwards) E.B.L.

—3,000 cc. Replaced blood 2,700 cc. I.V. fluids—D 5% H_2O—300 cc; N.S.—250 cc.

Under general anesthetic, in a dorsal recumbent position, chest, abdomen, and inguinal area were prepared with pHisoHex and tr. iodine and alcohol. Sterile drapes were applied. The chest was entered through a vertical sternal-splitting incision, and bleeding was controlled with electrocautery and bone wax.

The pericardium was incised vertically. Inspection of the heart revealed marked ventricular enlargement and marked dilatation of and tortuosity of the ascending aorta. The patient received 3 mg of heparin per kilo of body weight. A tube was placed in the right atrium and the left ventricle vented with a catheter. A catheter was placed in the ascending aorta for arterial infusion from the heart-lung machine. Extracorporeal circulation was instituted and the body temperature was reduced to 33°C. The aorta was cross-clamped and opened. The calcified, stenotic aortic valve was removed and replaced with a Starr-Edwards ball-valve prosthesis. Coronary arteries were perfused intermittently during the replacement. After the valve insertion, the aorta was closed with two layers of silk suture. Extracorporeal circulation was discontinued and the heart defibrillated with a single shock of 20 watt/sec. The ventricular vent was closed, the aortic cannula removed, and the aortotomy sutured. The chest was drained with two ⅜-inch tubes. Anatomic layers were closed with wire and silk suture. Dressings were applied. The condition of patient was "satisfactory."

The patient was on extracorporeal circulation for one hour and ten minutes. Medications during surgery were:

Heparin
Atropine
Mannitol
Innovar
Protamine
Calcium chloride
Prostigmin

Anes: Pentothal
Nitrous oxide oxygen
Muscle relaxant

Central venous pressure varied from 13½ to 21 cm. Blood pressure was 150/80 at the beginning of surgery and 120/70 at the close of surgery.

The lowest temperature during perfusion was 32⁵°C. At the close of surgery, it was 37°C.

Total operative time, 3¼ hr
Anes. time, 4 hr

Mr. Prince's venous and arterial blood was monitored for oxygen, carbon dioxide saturation bicarbonates, pH, and hemoglobin frequently in the operating room.

6/25/72—IMMEDIATE POSTOPERATIVE ORDERS

1. V.S. q. 15 min until stable then q. 1 h.
2. N.T. aspiration q. 1 h.
3. Observe chest drainage—milk chest tubes q.h., record hourly. If condition is good, sit up and cough, deep breathe q.h.
4. Report C.V.P. below 15, chest drainage over 250 cc/hr and urine output less than 20 cc/hr to M.D.
5. I.V.'s—500 cc D 5% H_2O c̄ 5 mu aqueous penicillin
   500 cc D 5% H_2O c̄ 5 mu aqueous penicillin
6. Drugs: Prostaphlin 1 g q. 4 h. via volutrol
   Streptomycin 500 mg q. 12 h. I.M.
7. Lab: C.B.C., fibrinogen, P.T.T., platelets, Hct., Hbg. at 8 P.M.
   C.B.C., BUN, Na, K, Cl, CO_2, Bilirubin, SGOT, platelets 1-3-5th P.O. Day.
   Daily Pro time
8. Chest x ray, EKG
9. Morphine sulphate 7 g q. 3–4 h. p.r.n. for pain
10. A.S.A. xx g q. 3–4 h. via suppository for temp. over 38.5°C.
    Blood C & S for temp. over 39°C.
11. IPPB c̄ N.S. for 15 min for 1 h then q. 4 h.
12. Weigh daily
13. Ice chips sparingly

The nurse caring for Mr. Prince in the intensive care unit received a brief résumé of Mr. Prince's surgery, blood loss, replacement, and condition in the operating room. When Mr. Prince arrived in the intensive care unit at 4:30 P.M., she noted the urinary output was 200 cc during his time in the operating room. She discarded this urine. Together with the anesthesiologist, she repositioned Mr. Prince, called him by name, and told him where he was. He responded by turning his head. The anesthesiologist removed the endotracheal tube. The two intravenous tubings, the central venous pressure tubing, and chest tubes were checked for patency. After Mr. Prince responded to his name, the head of the bed was elevated slightly.

Summary of Nurse's Observations

4:30–11:00 P.M.

Vital signs stable. Blood pressure varied from 120/80 to 140/90; pulse 80 to 100, fairly regular, peripheral pulses palpable; temperature 37.2°C at 6 P.M., 38°C at 11 P.M. Aspirin grains xx given by suppository; chest drainage 25 to 30 cc per hour, sero-sanguineous; urine output 30 to 75 cc per hour; central venous pressure varied from 15 to 24. Coughs well and productively. No need for suctioning. Monitor pattern—normal sinus rhythm.

Mrs. Prince visited every hour until 10 P.M. She was assured that his condition was satisfactory.

11:00–7:00 A.M.

Vital signs fairly stable. Apical pulse around 100 but more irregular. Monitor pattern—P waves missing several times a minute. Central venous pressure slowly from 24 to 13. Total intake since surgery 1,260 cc. Total output 1,560 cc. Urine 845, chest 715.

JUNE 26

8:00 A.M.

Mr. Prince had a restless night, but said he slept a few minutes "off and on." Central venous pressure 13. Weight 82.4 kg. Leaking blood around the chest tube. Dressings bright red, but not completely saturated. Medical staff notified. Chest film taken: negative, lungs clear, well aereated.

New I.V. orders: (1) 500 cc D 5% H_2O c̄ 5 mu aqueous penicillin
(2) 1,000 cc D 5% H_2O c̄ 5 mu aqueous penicillin
200 cc water—in sips.

Lab report: W.B.C. 11,200; platelets 122,000; urea N. 26, Ha 136, K 3.9, Cl 97, CO_2 31, Pro time: control 13.7, pt. 14.5.

8:00 A.M.

B.P. 158/88, pulse 72, temp. 38.3°C, central venous pressure 15. Chest drainage—none. Urine 30 cc.

12:00 noon

B.P. 136/70, pulse 100, central venous pressure 16.4. Urine output 12 to 25 cc per hour. No chest drainage since 8 A.M. Monitor pattern—irregularity—P waves missing. Mr. Prince is more restless and anxious, does not cough. Breath sounds difficult to hear. Apical pulse irregular. Medical staff notified of above observation. Mr. Prince continued to be restless all afternoon, but had no marked change in vital signs except central venous pressure was 13 and urine output averaged 15 cc per hour.

5:00 P.M.

B.P. 86/50, pulse 180, weak, thready, peripheral pulse not palpable. Skin clammy. Physician notified again. Mr. Prince was taken to the operating room for emergency exploratory sternotomy.

Mrs. Prince was notified of Mr. Prince's condition and that there was blood leaking, very likely from a large vessel.

Report of Surgery

D 5% and H_2O—1,000 cc

Blood replacement during surgery 1,500 cc

Blood loss 3,100 cc

Vigorous bleeding was encountered at the root of the aorta at the right medial side of the aortotomy. Resuturing with reinforcement of teflon pledgets of aorta.

Hemostasis was satisfactory.

Systolic blood pressure at beginning of surgery at 5:30 P.M., 50; 7:00 P.M.. 100; and at 8:00 P.M., 120.

Condition was termed satisfactory upon his return to the intensive care unit.

11:00 P.M.: hemoglobin 11.8, Hct. 35.

M.D. orders: Continue I.V. ordered this A.M. Resume post-op orders from last surgery.

NURSE'S ACTIONS

The nurse checked his temperature, which was 39°C; gave aspirin suppository ten grains. Chest drainage has clots, tubing milked frequently, 25 cm per hour. Ice bags to groin and axilla. Patient coughing and expectorating copiously. Patient is oriented, but very tired. Tachycardia pulse 116 all night.

JUNE 27

7:00 A.M.
Vital signs fairly stable. Temperature 38.0°C; B.P. 144/80 to 114/70; apical pulse 110+ and irregular; central venous pressure 15. to 11. Urinary output adequate, clear amber. Taking fluids orally. Weight 82.5 kg.

New Orders

Fluid orders same
Digoxin 0.5 mg q.i.d. after lead tt
Weight 81 kg

Nurse Notes

Mr. Prince rested and slept but was easily aroused. Continues to cough and expectorate copious brown secretion. Output adequate. Mr. Prince told Miss

Lee that he wished he were allowed to sleep more but "I guess they have to keep close watch." He is still fibrile. Foley and central venous pressure catheters removed. Urinary output adequate—color of urine, amber.

JUNE 29

Chest tube drainage—24 hr: 105 cc
Weight 79.9 kg
Total intake 24 hr 1,500 cc (1,000 cc I.V., 500 cc oral)
Output 1,250 cc (urinary and chest)
Dulcolax suppository with "good" results
Mr. Prince hiccoughed intermittently all day. These were relieved for a short period of time by using paper bag method of rebreathing.

Mr. Prince asked the physician if he could be transferred to his room downstairs, where he felt he could rest better and visit with his wife. The physician said he would remove his chest tube tomorrow and after that, if everything looked as well as today, he would be transferred.

JUNE 30

Weight 78.8 kg. Temperature 37.8°C.

I.V. therapy discontinued. Soft diet with 1,500 milligrams salt and fluid restriction to 1,500 cc.

Chest tube removed.

11:00 A.M.: Transferred to surgical unit. He coughs productively. Mr. Prince continued to hiccough. Paper bag breathing helps a short time.

JULY 1

Compazine 10 mg given several times during the night for hiccoughs. He had brief periods of relief.

Lab reports: Hbg. 10.7; Hct. 32.5; W.B.C. 13,060; platelets 304,000; Na 140; K 4.3; Cl 98; CO_2 31.

Because Mr. Prince's hemoglobin was low, he was given a preparation of ferrous sulphate 300 mg orally three times a day. Mr. Prince could be up and about as tolerated.

Mr. Prince told Miss Lee that he had to go to the bathroom that morning and the nurse found him and sure "bawled me out" for getting up without help. Mr. Prince's hiccoughs were relieved when he walked about. The hiccoughs resumed again, even at night. He used the paper bag frequently. At one visit, when Mr. Prince's hiccoughing was quite severe, Miss Lee sat down to talk about plans for going home and how he might manage. He knew already that he would be restricting fluids and salt and that his activity would be governed by shortness of breath. He said he could now sleep with the head of the bed lowered more than before. He also understood that he would be on iron pills until his hemoglobin was up, and this would give him more "pep." After about 20 minutes, Mr. Prince's hiccoughs stopped completely. Mr. Prince decided that the hiccoughs had some relation with his degree of tenseness and he felt more relaxed now. Phenobarbital 30 mg, Prostaphlin and streptomycin were resumed same as pre-operatively.

JULY 3

All antibiotics were discontinued. Temperature normal. Apical pulse 88, still irregular. Mr. Prince, although tiring easily after exertion, was in good spirits. He said he felt he would do well at home where he could sleep in familiar surroundings. Mr. Prince ate well and followed fluid restriction orders. He was still exercising and coughing and expectorating some.

Hiccoughing was less frequent. He felt now he could control hiccoughs himself by being in an upright position, taking very deep slow breaths, and rebreathing from a paper bag. He verbalized some fear that the stitches might open up his aorta again and this time he would not be so lucky. Miss Lee replied that the suturing of the aorta was more than adequate and very likely healing was progressing as expected. In talking with Mrs. Prince, Miss Lee assessed Mrs. Prince's understanding of her husband's changes in activity, salt and fluid restriction. Mrs. Prince was quite well informed and understood Mr. Prince's requirements. She felt that she needed to help Mr. Prince discipline himself to less taxing physical activity, because he had always been active before. She had experience preparing a low salt diet, but needed some further clarification. Both Mr. and Mrs. Prince were instructed to count his radial pulse. Miss Lee informed both about the toxic cumulative effects of digitoxin and what they needed to observe. Mr. Prince had occasional hiccoughs until the day of discharge on July 7. Vital signs range from 7/3/72 until 7/7/72 are as follows: temp. 36.5 to 37.5°C; apical pulse 84 to 110, still slightly irregular; B.P. range 104/68 to 128/90; weight 78 kg. Weight loss was 9.7 kg. since his hospital admission date in June.

Mr. Prince was instructed to see his local medical doctor weekly and to return to the outpatient clinic on August 14. A week after discharge, Mr. Prince had not gained weight, was beginning to enjoy food made with a salt substitute, and was taking walks in the yard, but with the extreme heat, he preferred to walk about the apartment. He said he had an opportunity to listen to his "new valve" and it "sure is loud and clear." He felt he could resume his usual job, with some curtailment of activities, after his "release" on August 14. The physician told Mr. Prince that he could do some supervision of janitorial work, but to wait for at least six weeks to resume any physical labor.

The public health nurse, who had received a referral from Miss Lee, visited Mr. Prince August 16 to assess Mr. Prince's progress and to evaluate Mr. and Mrs. Prince's understanding of his diet, salt restriction, exercise and rest regime. She found Mr. Prince had no leg edema and his weight remained at 78 kg. She also found Mr. Prince was scheduling activities succeeding his rest periods after meals. He was satisfied at this time that he had sufficient activity, but worried about getting back to work. His son and wife took over his janitorial activities under his supervision. Soon his son would be enrolled in school, but felt that he gradually could resume some activities and help his wife. He said he did not want his wife to work so hard, and janitorial work was not for a woman.

STUDY GUIDE

Preoperative Period

1. Describe the dynamics of congestive heart failure in Mr. Prince's case.
2. What is the difference between right-sided and left-sided failure?
3. Describe the therapeutic action of a low salt diet in Mr. Prince's case.
   a. Plan a liquid diet for a day allowing 1,500 mg salt and fluids restricted to 1,500 cc.
   b. Plan a regular diet with the same restrictions. How would you plan to distribute fluids?
4. After Mr. Prince was told he was to have a heart catheterization, he told the nurse he would rather go through another hernia operation than the impending catheterization. How would you, as a nurse, respond to Mr. Prince's statement?
5. Why is it important for the patient to learn before surgery how to exercise? To deep breathe? To cough?
6. How would you evaluate the patient's ability to do the above? Demonstrate.
7. Discuss the practice of routinely touring the I.C.U. with all preoperative heart patients.
8. What are the differences in action between digoxin and digitoxin? What is meant by digitalizing? What are the signs and symptoms of digitalis toxicity?
9. Why is it important for the nurse to assess the cardiopulmonary and vascular function before surgery?
10. Demonstrate palpation of extremity pulses.
11. What might be the status of the respiratory system after cardiac surgery?

12. What is the significance of the following lab tests in Mr. Prince's case: sodium, potassium, chloride, carbon dioxide, hemoglobin, hematocrit, blood urea nitrogen?
13. Describe the purpose and action of the preoperative medications.
    a. What are toxic actions of atropine?
    b. What are the differences in action between Scopolomine and atropine?
14. What is meant by "giving support" to the adult preoperative patient and his family?

Surgery

1. What is the action of heparin?
2. Why was CaCl given? Why was protamine given?
3. Mr. Prince's body temperature was lowered during extracorporeal circulation. Why?
4. Why were blood gases monitored during surgery?

Postoperative Period

A. *Fluid and electrolytes.* Why is maintenance of fluids and electrolyte balance so vital? What are nursing responsibilities?
   1. How is kidney perfusion evaluated?
   2. Of what value are central venous pressure readings? What is the importance of position of the patient and monometer during readings of C.V.P.?
   3. What intravenous fluids are used most frequently? Why?
   4. What are the dangers of overtransfusing?
   5. How and why record chest tube drainage?
   6. How significant is wound drainage in fluid balance?
B. *Vital signs.* Why is the taking of vital signs a necessary part of postoperative assessment?
   1. Discuss the accuracy of blood pressure readings in detecting postoperative complications such as shock and heart failure.
   2. In taking the apical, radial, and peripheral pulses, what must the nurse be alert for? Demonstrate palpation of lower extremity peripheral pulses.
   3. How does the nurse assess the efficiency of the internal and external respiratory system?
   4. What measures were taken with Mr. Prince to increase and maintain respiratory functioning?
   5. What signs indicated the onset of bleeding with Mr. Prince?

6. Discuss the actions of the nurse at this time.
7. Why is an elevated temperature a common occurrence following open-heart surgery?
8. What may have been the cause of Mr. Prince's arrhythmia?
C. What visual observations of the patient are necessary? Why?
D. Of what importance is positioning in maintaining cardiopulmonary function?
E. *Other complications.*
    1. What signs or symptoms may indicate neurological malfunction due either to organic pathology or psychological effects?
    2. What are signs of infection?
    3. What are nursing assessments in detection of postoperative infection? What is the nurse's responsibility in prevention of infection?
    4. How does a nurse determine activity level for a patient with heart disease?
F. Provision for comfort—physical and emotional
    1. What are the more common discomforts due either directly or indirectly from cardiac surgery?
    2. What nursing measures might be used?
    3. What may have caused Mr. Prince's hiccoughs (singultus)? What happens physiologically during hiccoughs? What is believed to be the action of carbon dioxide in relieving hiccoughs?
G. *Discharge planning.* Cardiac functional evaluation was done by the physician when the patient returned to the clinic. It was believed that Mr. Prince's cardiac status would gradually return to his pre-illness status. What kinds of specific instructions would you give Mr. and Mrs. Prince to facilitate his convalescence?

SELECTED READINGS

K. Andreoli, "The Cardiac Monitor," *American Journal of Nursing*, vol. 69, no. 6, June 1969, pp. 1238–1243.

C. Barnes, "Working with Parents of Children Undergoing Cardiac Surgery," *Nursing Clinics of North America*, vol. 4, no. 1, March 1969, pp. 11–18.

P. Barton, "Play as a Tool of Nursing," *Nursing Outlook*, vol. 10, March 1962, p. 162.

C. Betson, "Blood Gases," *American Journal of Nursing*, vol. 68, no. 5, May 1968, pp. 1010–1012.

C. Betson *et al.*, "Cardiac Surgery in Neonates, A Chance for Life," *American Journal of Nursing*, vol. 69, no. 1, January 1969, pp. 69–73.

L. Brunner *et al.*, "Patients with Conditions of the Heart," *Medical-Surgical Nursing*, J. B. Lippincott, Philadelphia, 1970, pp. 393–404.

G. C. Elliott and P. Winchell, "Heart Catheterization and Angiocardiography," *American Journal of Nursing*, vol. 60, October 1960, p. 1418.

F. Erickson, "Therapeutic Relationship of the Nurse to the Parents of a Sick Child," *Conference on Maternal and Child Nursing*, Ross Laboratories, Columbus, Ohio, 1965.

W. Ganong, *Medical Physiology*, Lange Medical Publications, Los Altos, California, 1969, chaps. 28–31, pp. 429–484; and chap. 33, pp. 502–515.

V. Hunn, "Cardiac Pacemakers," *American Journal of Nursing*, vol. 69, no. 4, April 1969, 749–754.

E. E. James, "The Nursing Care of the Open Heart Patient," *Nursing Clinics of North America*, (September 1967), pp. 543–557.

H. Mitchell *et al.*, *Cooper's Nutrition in Health and Disease*, 15th ed., 1968, pp. 327–341.

C. Moore and M. Rose, "Working with Children and Their Families to Help Them Through a Long-Anticipated Surgical Experience," from Betty Bergersen *et al.*, *Current Concepts in Clinical Nursing*, C. V. Mosby, St. Louis, 1967, pp. 311–327.

R. Peay, "The Emotional Problems of Children Facing Heart Surgery," *Children*, vol. 7, no. 6, November–December, 1960, pp. 223–228.

E. Pitorak *et al.*, *Nurse's Guide to Cardiac Surgery and Nursing Care*, McGraw-Hill, New York, 1969.

E. Pitorak, "Open-Ended Care for the Open Heart Patient," *American Journal of Nursing*, vol. 67, July 1967, pp. 1452–1457.

W. Reed and J. Yokes, "Heart Surgery," Lawrence Meltzer *et al.* (ed.), *Concepts and Practice of Intensive Care*, Charles Press, Philadelphia, 1969, pp. 374–392.

B. Rogos, "Nursing Care of the Cardiac Surgery Patient," *Nursing Clinics of North America*, vol. 4, no. 4, December 1969, pp. 631–644.

H. Shields, "Cardiac Anatomy and Physiology," *Nursing Clinics of North America*, vol. 4, no. 4, December 1969, pp. 563–572.

B. Smith, "Congestive Heart Failure," *American Journal of Nursing*, vol. 69, no. 2, (February 1969), pp. 278–282. Three treatment goals are described: Reducing patient's requirements for oxygen, elimination of edema, and increased cardiac output.

S. Williams, *Nutrition and Diet Therapy, Cardio-Vascular Disease*, 1st ed., C. V. Mosby, St. Louis, 1969, pp. 528–535.

Mrs. Simon
fifty-eight years old

Diabetes Mellitus and Leg Amputation/Chronic
Margaret Peterson

In 1968, a home care unit was a part of the University of Kansas Medical Center under the direction of the Department of Preventive Medicine. The team approach to giving patient care in the home was used with students from medicine, nursing, physical therapy, occupational therapy, and nutrition, as well as a social worker.

Assessment of the patient's needs and desires for home care was made by this multidisciplinary team while the patient was in the hospital. Goals were set up with the patient and his family. A referral was made through the hospital community health coordinator to the home care unit, and prior to discharge, an evaluation visit was made to the home by the team. The team then gave direct care to the patient and the patient's family in the home. Mrs. Simon and her family were one of these families.

NURSING HISTORY

Mrs. Simon is a fifty-eight-year-old female with diabetes mellitus, congestive heart failure, and a mid-thigh amputation of the right leg. She has been known to this hospital since 1948.

Mrs. Simon and her husband live in a fourteen-room home in a low-middle-class neighborhood. She feels that she was a perfectionist and it "bothered" her if the house was not "proper" at all times. She has two sons and one daughter who were all married and living near the family home. She also has eighteen grandchildren. Her husband is seventy-four years old and works as a janitor in a department store. Mrs. Simon receives Social Security for her disability, and with her husband's salary and the rent, they are financially independent.

Mrs. Simon was born in Tennessee, one of seven children. Her formal education was limited to two or three years; however, she is able to read and write to some degree. She feels what her mother taught her in childhood had a direct bearing on her ability to walk with a prosthesis and to return to activities of daily living. She said her mother taught her "to do what we were doing and to do it right" and so she wanted to walk "right." This attitude no doubt helped her determination to walk well on the prosthesis. Mrs. Simon was usually an uncomplaining and accepting person. Even with her loss of a leg and problems in ambulation, her self-image did not seem to change. However, during the period of two months when she had three amputations, she was prone to depression. She was quite apprehensive, as was manifested by her irritable and complaining behavior. She had difficulty in directly communicating these anxieties and depended heavily on her daughter's strengths to comfort her.

This is a closely knit family unit. The patient's children are vitally interested in her, and her daughter took a considerable amount of responsibility in promoting health care and giving emotional support. She also took her to clinic appointments.

Before the episodes which terminated in a series of leg amputations, Mrs. Simon had been actively involved in the community and especially in local church affairs. She had taken care of her home and had been active in keeping the family structure strong and cohesive. She also felt she had maintained a regular regimen in the care of her diabetes. Her neighborhood, clubs, lodge, and church gave her much emotional support and encouragement during her hospitalization. Also, they contributed money to help her buy the prosthesis. This became such a "precious commodity" that both Mrs. Simon and her husband did not want to use it.

MEDICAL-SURGICAL HISTORY AND TREATMENT

Mrs. Simon had been comparatively well until 1947, when it was discovered she had diabetes. She had a "blackout" and fell on the street. She was taken to a local hospital for treatment. She was told by a doctor that she had diabetes, must follow a certain diet, and take insulin every day. According to Mrs. Simon, she had been given no specific instructions on the diet or how to take insulin injections. This was an emotional crisis in her life. She said she had no knowledge of the consequences of inadequate diabetic care. Shortly thereafter, she seemed to "feel better" and discontinued taking her insulin. In 1949, she was hospitalized for uterine fibroids, and at that time she was again instructed to take insulin. On pages 208–209 is a résumé, taken from the charting of her medical and surgical treatment to the time she was dismissed to the multidisciplinary team for care.

NURSING AND TEAM PROCESS

As we review Mrs. Simon's history and need for an amputation, we ask what might have been done, if anything, to avoid these complications.

In 1965, foot care was an imminent need. She had given evidence of this in 1963. Upon obtaining the nursing history from Mrs. Simon, the "noncompliance" label, given her in December 1965, took on new meaning. She explained that there had been a great deal of financial difficulty, as well as the fact transportation for them was practically an impossibility. Therefore, she could not attend clinic as suggested.

In February of 1966, she had an added diagnosis of congestive heart failure. It would have seemed advantageous at this point for a referral to have been made to monitor both the heart condition and the diabetes. The home care unit nutritionist would have been an asset in teaching the 1,400 calorie diet. To understand the cultural patterns of food and eating is an important factor in helping plan a good diet. One of the important nursing functions with patients who have congestive heart failure is to recognize the activities that may increase work for the heart. With scheduled home visits, these are often brought under control before decompensation begins.

The multidisciplinary team, during the period from August 1967 to September 1968, made periodic home visits, planning with Mrs. Simon her activities of daily living.

As noted in the introduction, a home visit was made prior to Mrs. Simon's discharge from the hospital. The purpose of the visit was to determine the level of activity that she might attain in the confines of her home; i.e., number of steps to climb to enter the home and how to get to the bathroom (note home safety evaluation chart). Mrs. Simon's goals, expressed to the nurse, were to return to her household tasks and to continue her church activities. These became the team's goals as well. To attain them, Mrs. Simon needed good nutrition, good walking habits with and without the prosthesis, and an understanding of her normal energy output. With goals established, the problems that were barriers to these goals had to be identified.

PROBLEM: DIABETES

When discharged from the hospital in February of 1967, Mrs. Simon had been told to take NPH Insulin at home. It was discovered, when checked in the home by the nurse (when the team began visiting in August of 1967), that she had been taking Lente Insulin for some time, as her husband would take an empty insulin bottle to the drugstore and purchase a similar one.

In December, her insulin dosage was changed to Regular 10 units (U 80) (short action) and NPH 35 units (U 80) (long action). Mrs. Simon needed

Date		Blood Sugar mg	Amount of Insulin units	Weight kg	Diet
Jan. 1949	Uterine fibroids.	206	Unknown	70	Carbohydrate 160 g Protein 80 g Fat 80 g
1963	A small ulcer developed on her foot following irritation by a nail in her shoe. She had a successful recovery except for a residual numbness on the bottom of her right foot.				
Dec. 1965	She was admitted to Kansas University Medical Center having an infected hypotrophic right great toe nail. She was discharged after the infection was controlled and advised to return to podiatry clinic. She was unable to get to clinic (the doctors labelled her as non-compliant).	298	Unknown	63.6	
Feb. 1966	She was diagnosed as having early congestive heart failure.	160	Unknown	65.5	1,400 calorie diabetic
May 1966	The great toe on the right foot was "black" under the nail. She had an upper respiratory infection.	324	Lente 55	65.9	1,400 calorie diabetic
Dec. 1966	She had a tack in her shoe. Cellulitis developed in her right leg and an ulcer under her foot.				
Dec. 31, 1966	2nd, 3rd and 4th toes on the right foot were amputated. Later, at the time of this hospitalization, the bottom of the right foot was darkening proximal to the amputation site. Diabetes was uncontrolled and the urine glucose was 4+.	342	Lente 55		
Jan. 10, 1967	A below-knee amputation was performed due to extensive cellulitis. She had symptoms of congestive heart failure. Patient was digitalized.				

Date	Notes				
Jan. 23, 1967	She attempted crutch walking, but there was a gaping wound and the stump was not healing. She fell out of bed when she was dreaming, injured the stump, and the wound became infected.	411	Insulin given on a sliding scale		
Feb. 6, 1967	An above-knee amputation was performed. The wound healed successfully. She attempted crutch walking with extreme fear of falling.	252	N.P.H. 45		
Aug. 1967	She was fitted with a prosthesis. Her husband said he used up his savings to get the $500 prosthesis and in paying the hospital bill. He also was afraid that she would fall while wearing the prosthesis. Both Mr. and Mrs. Simon had negative attitudes in using the prosthesis. At this time the team began their home visits.	342	N.P.H. 40	50.4	
Nov. 1967	Chest pain returned with increased ambulation. Digitalis and nitroglycerin were given.	429	N.P.H. 55	55 with prosthesis	
Dec. 1967	The physician reported that because of questionable angina and other vascular disease, it was probably better that she not be subjected to hypoglycemic episodes and best that she have at least + trace of sugar in her urine most of the time.	306	Reg 10 N.P.H. 35	55	1,500 calories
Feb. 1968	She increased her ambulation and was using parallel bars in the home to increase her performance.	435	Reg 15 N.P.H. 38		
Sept. 1968	Mrs. Simon is wearing her prosthesis. She uses the cane periodically and is able to ambulate wherever she wants to go. There have been no further symptoms of congestive heart failure, but she continues her digitalis medication. The diabetes, as shown by the fluctuating blood sugar, remains a problem.				

instructions in administering this properly. Practice sessions were held by the nurse to increase her confidence. It was difficult for her to change her habit of drawing the plunger of the syringe from the 55 mark to the 45 mark. A tape was put on the syringe to remind her. Even though patients may have had diabetes for a period of time, we cannot be sure they remember all the instructions. Continual assessment and reeducation are necessary. Explanations were given regarding insulin actions and the necessity to continue her diet. The team nutritionist was asked to reassess and further instruct on diet.

Even though Mrs. Simon had had diabetes for several years, it was necessary to teach the rudiments of a maintenance regime. To be able to do this in her own home was an advantage to the nurse, as well as to the patient. Urine testing was again explained. The use of the clinitest was reiterated. Mrs. Simon had not thought this important. Bottles of old clinitest tape were found in the bathroom closet.

Mrs. Simon was well aware of the necessity of foot care. Teaching on this point was just to remind her of cleanliness to the foot, about wearing the right kind of shoe and hose, and to watch her toes for any corn or callus. She was also told the danger of sudden cold and heat changes.

Mrs. Simon's attitude to this information was one of appreciation, and she made foot care a part of her activities of daily living.

PROBLEM: AMBULATION AND EXERCISE

The nurse consulted with the physical therapist and the occupational therapist regarding the safety check and the household activities performance test (see enclosure).

HOME SAFETY EVALUATION CHART

NAME_____DATE_____

ADDRESS_____PHONE NUMBER_____

DISABILITY_____

HOUSE_____APARTMENT_____LIVE ALONE_____

Access to Living Area:

Elevator_____ Steps_____ Well Lighted?_____

Bannisters or hand railing_____ Sidewalks_____ Ramp_____

General Household:

1. Doorways: Number of outside doors_____ Inside doorways_____
   Wide enough for wheel chair_____

2. Floors: Slippery_____ Free of clutter_____
   Throw rugs anchored_____ or removed_____
   Linoleum free of hole and rough places_____

3. Furniture: Sturdy_____ Equipped with coasters_____
   Arranged for free movement_____

4. Electrical and telephone cords: Not in traffic pattern_____
   no overloaded circuits_____ work areas well lighted_____

5. Storage areas: Free of clutter_____ easily accessible_____

6. Heating system: Stove located where not hazardous_____
   Central_____ Radiators_____

Bathroom:

Rails for tub_____ Toilet_____
Non-slip mats in tub and/or shower_____
Medicines clearly labeled_____ Stored at bedside_____

Kitchen:

Stove—Burner controls easily accessible_____
Lightweight pots and pans_____ Heavy potholder or mitts_____
Adequate counter space close to stove_____
Faucets—Easily accessible_____ mixer type_____
Use wheeled cart or basket to transport dishes, clothes, etc._____

Bedroom:

Bed arranged so easy to get in and out of_____
Trapeze_____ Hospital bed_____ Other_____

Bedroom:

Closet easily accessible —————————————————————————————

Night light in bedroom/bathroom area and in hall————————————————

Flashlight available—————————————————————————————————

Comments: (include additional equipment needed)

———

———

———

———

Teaching was an important means of helping Mrs. Simon toward independence. With the strong and warm family relationship, there was a tendency on the part of her husband and children not to allow her to do things for herself. This proved to be a difficulty in helping her toward her independent role again.

Originally, the husband had kept the patient from wearing the prosthesis. He had a fear that she would fall, either hurting herself or breaking the artificial limb. He had stayed away from his work to care for her. He had done the cooking and performed the various household tasks. He had returned to work when Mrs. Simon was able to use the wheelchair, but would phone her several times a day, much to her irritation. Indignantly she stated, "I can get around by myself now—he doesn't need to worry about me."

The husband was included in determining how furniture should be placed in order that the wheelchair could be used. He helped in firming rugs on the floor. They both heard explanations on proper use of the prosthesis by the physical therapist. He insisted in putting up temporary parallel bars to give Mrs. Simon more exercise. As she progressed, she could use crutches and walker, and finally was able to ambulate on her prosthesis with a cane. Many older persons do not have the balance and coordination necessary for walking properly.

PROBLEM: TO BE ABLE TO FULFILL HER ROLE AS HOMEMAKER

To cook, wash dishes, iron, and make the beds were Mrs. Simon's goals. The occupational therapist was consulted and a check list was used to determine her level of functioning. Various kitchen utensils were placed for her convenience and a stool was provided for her to rest upon for washing dishes and ironing.

Several disciplines are needed in the rehabilitation of an amputee. Close professional relationships among members of the team who contributed knowledge from different disciplines was essential to ensure effective assessment, teaching, and rehabilitation of Mrs. Simon.

Mrs. Simon, at first, was self-conscious in wearing the artificial limb in public. She also had a fear of falling when she wore the limb. However, she had a great desire to return to church. The occupational therapist, physical therapist, and nurse made an evaluation of what might be architectural barriers to prevent her from going to church. There were unlevel sidewalks on which she must learn to walk and there were steps up to enter the church. She was taught how to walk on the sidewalk and how to get into the car. There was a side door to the church on the ground level. It was suggested she leave for church early, go through the side door, and get seated before the people came. Mrs. Simon responded to these suggestions and on a subsequent visit she said, "Now I am where I want to be." Later she was able to walk to the grocery store with her husband and do her shopping—another one of her goals.

CONCLUSION

Mrs. Simon was told she could control her diabetes fairly well and thus lead a normal life. She had learned the necessity of good skin care and accepted this as a part of life in her daily pattern of activities. Her eating habits were stabilized and her former insatiable desire for sweets had diminished.

She returned as an active member of society. She did not return to her former speed of activities, but she maintained her home, was a strength again in the family unit, and was a participating member of her church.

She responded well to rehabilitation following amputation. Her diabetes remained brittle, but she returned frequently to the diabetic clinic. Her arteriosclerotic heart disease was essentially asymptomatic. She took digitalis and occasionally nitroglycerin. She was taught, by the student nurse, to notice any signs of digitalis intoxication.

Sir William Osler stated, "To live a long life is to contract a chronic disease and take care of it." Mrs. Simon was doing just that at the point of termination of the visits by the home care team. She had moved from dependence to independence and self-care. We utilized the teaching, guiding, counseling continuum by telling, explaining, and directing her toward independence, using the expertise of the nurse and the other health discipline members together with the strengths of the family. Nursing and the other health disciplines labeled this family situation as a "success story."

STUDY GUIDE

1. Discuss the signs and symptoms of diabetes and its natural history. Compare the adult and juvenile types of diabetes.
2. What means are used in the early detection of diabetes? What are the diagnostic measures?
3. What circulatory complications may be affected by diabetes and what are some of the untoward results?
4. If a person has diabetes, what are the acute complicating factors, i.e., how would you differentiate symptoms of hypoglycemia and diabetic acidosis?
5. What do you consider in teaching a person with diabetes about insulin, urine testing, personal hygiene, exercise, and diet?
6. What are the problems in counseling a person with diabetes; i.e., in pregnancy and family planning, in homemaking, and in the environment?
7. What nursing care should be given a patient before and after an amputation?
8. What does a nurse need to know to help a patient walk with crutches and/or with an artificial leg?
9. How would you, as a nurse, coordinate efforts of other people in your community to assist those with physical handicaps or those in a situation like Mrs. Simon's?
10. Discuss the home visit in relation to patient care and family teaching.

SELECTED READINGS

Helen M. Arnold, "Elderly Diabetic Amputee," *American Journal of Nursing,* December 1969, pp. 2646–2649.

Ruth Freeman, *Community Health Nursing Practice,* W. B. Saunders, Philadelphia, 1970, chap. 8, pp. 120–133.

James F. Garret and Edna S. Levine, *Psychological Practices with the Physically Disabled,* Colorado University Press, 1966, pp. 1–46.

Lydia Halley, "The Physical Therapist: Who, What and How," *American Journal of Nursing,* July 1970, pp. 1521–1524.

Effie Hanchett and Ruth Johnson, "Early Signs of Congestive Heart Failure," *American Journal of Nursing,* July 1968, pp. 1456–1461.

Jean E. Holmes, "The Physical Therapist and Team Care," *Nursing Outlook,* March 1972, pp. 182–184.

May Hornback, "Diabetes Mellitus—The Nurse's Role," *The Nursing Clinics of North America,* W. B. Saunders, Philadelphia, March 1970, pp. 3–11.

Merry Chellas (ed.), "Insulin Reactions in a Brittle Diabetic," *Nursing '72*, May 1972, pp. 6–11.

Carroll B. Larson and Marjorie Gould, *Orthopedic Nursing*, 7th ed., C. B. Mosby, St. Louis, 1970, pp. 434–450.

Eli Lily, *Diabetes Mellitus*, 7th ed., Lily Research Laboratories, Indianapolis, 1967, pp. 87–109, 159–164.

Donna Nickerson, "Teaching the Hospitalized Diabetic," *American Journal of Nursing*, May 1972, pp. 935–938.

Ruth W. Spain, "Rehabilitative Nursing," *The Nursing Clinics of North America*, September 1966, pp. 355–362.

Sarah Stuart, "Day to Day Living with Diabetes," *American Journal of Nursing*, August 1971, pp. 1548–1550.

Mr. Moore
sixty-five years old

Cataract/Chronic
Lucille D. Gress

INTRODUCTION

The most common disability that occurs in the aged eye as a result of the normal aging process is cataract formation or opacity of the lens. Frequently aged individuals with cataractous lens are a part of the population of the eye, ear, nose, and throat unit of the medical center hospital. Mr. Moore is an example of the aged family member experiencing a crisis episode precipitated by cataract formation in his right eye. The decrease in visual acuity caused a disruption of equilibrium resulting in the need for medical treatment and for nursing intervention.

GENERAL DESCRIPTION

Mr. Moore is a somewhat obese, ambulatory sixty-five-year-old retired mine worker with greying hair and a receding hair line. He is outgoing and a reliable historian. His chief complaint on admission to the hospital: "Cataract on my right eye."

PRESENT MEDICAL HISTORY

There has been a gradual decrease in visual acuity (VA) in the right eye (OD). No decrease of VA in the left eye (OS), although Mr. Moore has been informed that there is cataract formation in the OS also. Previous physical examination three years ago. No history or evidence of diabetes mellitus.

Vital Signs.   Blood pressure 120/80, temperature 36.7°C, pulse 72, respiration 18; height 5 feet, 10 inches, weight 80.3 kg.

Diagnosis.   Cataract, right eye.

Treatment.   Cataract extraction, right eye.

PAST MEDICAL HISTORY

Mr. Moore's medical history included information about "stomach trouble" that he sometimes experiences at night and an account of an allergic reaction to penicillin (hives). Maalox relieves the gastric distress. Otherwise, the findings of previous physical examinations are essentially normal.

SOCIAL HISTORY

Mr. Moore lives with his wife in a small town 80 miles from the medical center. He retired 1½ years ago and receives a pension from the United Mine Workers. Insurance coverage includes that from the United Mine Welfare Fund and Medicare. His wife, sixty-two years of age, recently began drawing social security benefits from her account established through her work as a secretary. The Moores have a high school education. Their religious affiliation is with the Reorganized Church of Jesus Christ of Latter Day Saints. The Moores share common interests in many areas, i.e., remodeling their home, attending auctions, fishing, traveling, and participating in senior citizen's activities. Mr. Moore spends some time in his woodworking shop.

Frequent visits with their married son, his wife and five granddaughters, who live in a nearby town, are a source of pleasure for the Moores. At one point, Mr. Moore said some people feel sorry for him because he does not have a grandson. "But," he added, "I've always liked the girls, especially my wife. We've been married forty-seven years."

DAILY HABITS

Mr. Moore reports that he used to be an early riser but now the usual "getting up time" tends to be approximately 7 A.M. This allows time for eliminating and shaving before becoming involved with other planned activities of the day. Mealtimes are fairly regular, 8 A.M., 12 noon, and 6 P.M. Mr. Moore says he has few vices. He does not smoke, but often takes a "sip of wine" at bedtime, usually 10 P.M. He enjoys card games and an occasional game of checkers, but is not interested in golfing or other more active sports. He and his wife try to plan activities to provide variation and adequate time for rest.

ADMISSION LABORATORY REPORTS

URINALYSIS	BLOOD COUNT	BLOOD SUGAR
7.5 pH	13.1 g percent hemoglobin	1 hr postprandial blood glucose 118 mg percent
1.001 specific gravity	42.3 hematocrit	
Protein negative	8,300 white blood cells	
Glucose negative	68 neutrophils	
1 + bacteria	4 monocytes 4 eosinophils adequate platelets	

NURSING ASSESSMENT

Nursing assessment is a means of identifying problems or needs of the patient/ family as a precursor to nursing intervention. In this case, a developmental focus is desirable, and, assessment should be on both the patient and family level. The framework of crisis theory provides another theoretical approach that indicates the need for assessing the coping ability of the patient/family during the crisis episode and the adaptation process that follows.

Mr. Moore and his wife are in the final developmental phase of the life cycle. They are experiencing disruption of their life style because of Mr. Moore's impairment of visual acuity. Indication of the level of coping ability is evident in the outreach for help with the problem. They are still able to function effectively, in spite of anxiety over the outcome of treatment. This ability should be useful in working through the adaptation process.

The long-term objective is to assist the Moores to work toward the goal of maximizing their potential for continuing development. This requires specific assessment of the family dynamics, of their knowledge and understanding of the problem, and their expectations of the proposed surgical treatment for Mr. Moore. Impairment of vision is a threat to the integrity of the family, as well as the integrity of the affected family member. This threat often engenders a high level of anxiety that may interfere with the course of treatment and rehabilitation process.

Since stress related to loss of vision may lead to behavioral change in the individual, i.e., disorientation, assessment of Mr. Moore's mental status is appropriate. The mental status questionnaire (M.S.Q.), or modification of it, may be used for the assessment. Hearing acuity should be noted in the initial interview in further assessment of a sensory deficit that is common in the aging person. Assessment of Mr. Moore's ability to carry out activities of daily living in the hospital should also be ascertained in the initial interaction.

NURSING DIAGNOSIS

1. The Moores are experiencing an increased level of anxiety related to hospitalization and concern over the outcome of the anticipated surgical procedure for cataract extraction for Mr. Moore.
2. Mr. Moore has impairment of vision that requires attention to safety factors and assistance with psychological aspects.
3. The Moores have educational needs in relation to the proposed plan of care and treatment.
4. There is need for mutual planning for continuity of care to facilitate rehabilitation and transfer from hospital to the home environment.

Plan

1. Begin to establish rapport with the Moores.
2. Orient the Moores to the hospital routines and environment.
3. Encourage expression of feelings and questions about their concerns.
4. Provide an appropriate environment in terms of limitations imposed by Mr. Moore's visual impairment.
5. Provide for preoperative care and teaching.
6. Provide for postoperative care and teaching.
7. Involve the Moores in planning for continuity of care.

Priorities

1. Establish rapport with the objective of decreasing the level of anxiety.
2. Orient the Moores to the hospital environment.
3. Explore the Moores's perception of their problem.
4. Begin the preoperative care and teaching.
5. Provide a safe environment.
6. Initiate discussion of the home situation as a precursor to planning for continuity of care.
7. Postoperativ ly, continue care and teaching.
8. Plan for continuity of care and initiate action to facilitate dismissal and the transfer to the home environment.

Medical Orders (Preoperative)

1. Diet as tolerated. Reg.
2. Nothing by mouth after midnight

3. C.B.C., U.A. serology, blood sugar
4. Neosporin Ophthalmic Solution drops 2 (right eye) 5, 7, 8, 9 P.M. the evening before surgery.
5. Benadryl 50 mg P.O. p.r.n. h.s.—may repeat once
6. Librium 15 mg P.O. 1½ hr pre-op
7. Vespirin 10 mg I.M. 1 hr pre-op day of surgery
8. Demerol 50 mg I.M. on call to O.R.
9. Neosynephrine 2½% Ophthalmic Solution drops 2 (right eye) q. 15 min. x4 starting 1½ hr pre-op on day of surgery.
10. Tap water or Fleets enema h.s. p.r.n.
11. A.S.A. 0.6 g (10 grains) 2 to 4 hr p.r.n.

6/15—SURGERY

Anesthetic: Local by retrobulbar injection

Intracapsular cataract extraction: Right eye

Irridectomy: Peripheral

Complications: None

Medical Orders (Postoperation)

1. Diet as tolerated
2. Demerol 50 mg I.M. q. 4–6 h. p.r.n. for pain
3. A.S.A. 0.6 g 10 grains q. 4 h. p.r.n. for pain
4. Darvon 65 mg q. 2–4 h. p.r.n. for pain
5. Benadryl 50 mg h.s. p.r.n. may repeat once
6. Vespirin 10 mg I.M. p.r.n. for nausea and restlessness
7. MOM 30 cc p.r.n. daily
8. Tap water or Fleets enema p.r.n. daily
9. May be up with help after 4 hr
10. Head of bed may be elevated to 90 degrees
11. May shave and gently comb hair on first P.O. day

PATIENT RESPONSE (ADMISSION, PREOPERATIVELY, POSTOPERATIVELY)—NURSE'S NOTES

6/14   12:00 P.M.
Ambulatory. Admitted to Room 349. Wife here.

12:45 P.M.
Senile and forgetful. Very nervous and talkative. Regular diet. Seemed to have difficulty understanding directions.

6:00 P.M.
Very talkative, appears confused. Answers to questions inappropriate. Urine specimen not sent (spilled specimen on floor).

8:00 P.M.
Urine specimen to lab.

6/15   *7:30* A.M.
Preparation started for surgery.

8:50 A.M.
Pupil of right eye dilated. Preoperative meds given. To surgery.

9:18 A.M.
Received in surgery, anesthetic—local.
Returned to floor/cart upon completion of the surgical procedure.

10:50 A.M.
Received in 349 East. Placed in bed, supine position, head of bed flat. Water given. No complaints.

12:50 P.M.
Restless. Complains of headache and nausea. Medication given. Surgical liquid lunch taken.

2:00 P.M.
Has been sleeping. Says he still has headache.

3:00 P.M.
Sleeping. Has not been up yet.

6:00 P.M.
Supper—ate fair.

9:00 P.M.
Ambulated to bathroom with assistance. Voided. No medication for sleep taken.

6/16   *6:00* A.M.
A good postoperative night. No complaints. Up to bathroom with assistance.

6/18—DAY OF DISMISSAL—CONVERSATION WITH THE NURSE THE DAY OF DISMISSAL

Mr. Moore said he guessed he was not worried about his eye because he knew he had one in reserve. He also said, "Sometimes you worry and don't know you're worrying." He attributed his uneventful recovery to a good attitude about his surgery and trust in his physician's competence. He said the doctor had told him there was no need to have the cataract extraction prior to retirement because of the kind of work he was doing. He also told him the dust would interfere with the use of a contact lens. Mr. Moore decided to have the surgery post-retirement hoping to "see better" so he and his wife can continue doing "what we've always wanted to do." As he referred to being fitted with a contact lens he said, "I'll do O.K., adjust to it."

ADAPTATION—PATIENT/FAMILY

Mr. Moore's recovery was uneventful. However, he verbalized that he sometimes worried without realizing it. His wife continued to be supportive during the postoperative period displaying a calm, quiet manner.

The Moores were anxious to leave for home the day of dismissal. They had Mr. Moore's personal belongings packed early. Mr. Moore sat on the edge of the bed "fidgeting" rather nervously as they waited for the prescription for ophthalmic medications to be filled and for the clinic appointment to be made.

Both expressed appreciation for Mr. Moore's care and for the help they received regarding his home care. Mrs. Moore said she was glad she knew how to drive the car, since it looked as if she would be the chauffeur for a while.

HOSPITAL PROGRESS

Uneventful postoperative course following cataract extraction, O.D. afebrile.

CONTINUITY OF CARE

Instructions were given for a return appointment to the clinic in one week. An instruction card for home care was presented to Mr. Moore with an explanation to him and his wife. The Moores were reminded that Mr. Moore should avoid strain on the suture line in his eye. Sudden movements, such as stooping to pick up an object off the floor or to tie shoes should be avoided. Constipation and straining of the stool should also be avoided.

DISMISSAL INSTRUCTIONS (ON CARD)

1. Do not rub or bump eye.
2. Wear colored glasses or your own glasses with operated eye lens blocked out during the day.
3. Wear metal shield at night, put on with scotch tape.
4. Two or three ophthalmic atropine (red top bottle) drops in operated eye 1 or 2 times a day. If more drops enter the eye, it will not damage the eye
5. Instill ¼ to ½ in. of Maxitrol ointment at bedtime (optional).

6. Use aspirin, Anacin, Bufferin, etc. for pain.
7. Wipe discharge from lids with cotton moistened with tap water daily. DO NOT PUT PRESSURE ON EYE.
8. Return to clinic 6/27/72 at 9 A.M.

STUDY GUIDE

1. What is a "senile" cataract? How does the cataract formation relate to the anatomy and physiology of vision?
2. In what ways may the developmental tasks of the aged individual and his family be disrupted by the formation of the "senile" cataract?
3. What are pertinent questions to be asked of the patient/family in the initial interview?
4. What are the important points of nursing care preoperatively?
5. What complications may arise postoperatively? What are the implications for nursing care?
6. What are the teaching/learning needs?
7. What approach should be used in providing for continuity of care?
8. What are the implications for nursing care of patients with sensory deprivation?
9. What principles of geriatric nursing may be used in the nurse/patient/family interaction?

SELECTED READINGS

J. Chodil and B. Williams, "The Concept of Sensory Deprivation," *Nursing Clinics of North America*, vol. 5, no. 3, W. B. Saunders, Philadelphia, September 1970, pp. 453–465.

E. D. Condl, "Ophthalmic Nursing: The Gentle Touch," *Nursing Clinics of North America*, vol. 5, no. 3, W. B. Saunders, Philadelphia, September 1970, pp. 467–476.

E. V. Cowdry, ed., *The Care of the Geriatric Patient*, 3rd ed., C. V. Mosby, St. Louis, 1968, pp. 25–26, 272–274.

I. C. Cullin, "Techniques for Teaching Patients with Sensory Defects," *Nursing Clinics of North America*, vol. 5, no. 3, W. B. Saunders, Philadelphia, September 1970, pp. 527–538.

C. W. Jackson, Jr., and R. Ellis, "Sensory Deprivation as a Field of Study," *Nursing Research*, vol. 20, no. 1, January–February 1971, pp. 46–54.

A. L. Karnzweig, "The Eye in Old Age," *Clinical Geriatrics*, Isadore Rossman, ed., J. B. Lippincott, Philadelphia, 1971, pp. 229–230.

L. Linn *et al.*, "Behavioral Disturbances Following Cataract Extraction," *American Journal of Psychiatry*, vol. 110, no. 281, 1953.

K. Newton and H. C. Anderson, *Geriatric Nursing*, 4th ed., C. V. Mosby, St. Louis, 1966, pp. 338–345, 347–348.

M. I. Ohno, "The Eye Patched Patient," *American Journal of Nursing*, vol. 71, no. 2, February 1971, pp. 271–274.

L. Schwartz and J. L. Schwartz, *The Psychodynamics of Patient Care*, Prentice-Hall, Englewood Cliffs, N.J., 1972, pp. 322–340.

Review anatomy and physiology of the eye.

Refer to a pharmacology text for information on medications.

Mr. Dice
sixty-five years old

Dissecting Abdominal Aortic Aneurysm/Acute
Judith A. Caudle

PATIENT PROFILE

Mr. Dice, sixty-five years old, was sweeping the floor at the elementary school in a small town when he suddenly stopped and grabbed his side. He was experiencing a very sharp stabbing pain in his right groin. He hurried to the custodian's room and lay down on the cot. When the pain didn't subside after an hour's rest, he became concerned and notified his local doctor. His local doctor, on examination of Mr. Dice found a large pulsating mass in the right lower quadrant. Mr. Dice was transferred to a medical center with a diagnosis of dissecting abdominal aortic aneurysm.

SOCIAL HISTORY

Mr. Dice and his wife came to the medical center together. Two of Mr. Dice's three daughters were unable to come with him since they were married and had families of their own to care for. However, Mr. Dice's youngest daughter did come to be with her mother and father as soon as she arranged for a replacement at her work.

Mr. Dice's job is being held open by the school district until he is able to return to work. The elementary school sent flowers to Mr. Dice. Mr. Dice has a very pleasant manner, but is very apprehensive since he has had no previous hospitalizations.

MEDICAL HISTORY

Mr. Dice is a tall, heavy Caucasian male with sharp abdominal pain of six hours duration. He denies having leg claudication or night cramping; has had no previous illness; and states he lives a quiet life with few hobbies and experiences no medical problems; has smoked two packs of Camels per day for 45 years.

PERTINENT PHYSICAL FINDINGS

1. Blood pressure 160/84
2. Pulse 84
3. Respirations 16
4. Grade ii arteriosclerotic changes of both fundi
5. Pulsatile mass covering entire right lower quadrant

LABORATORY STUDIES

Complete blood count showing an increase in white blood cells. Urinalysis was within normal limits.
Type and cross match for 10 units of blood
Blood urea nitrogen 20 mg %
Serum creatinine 1.5 mg %
Serum electrolytes: Na 132, K 3.9, Cl 110, CO_2 content 20
Electrocardiogram within normal limits
Prothrombin time within normal limits

The x ray showed calcification of the abdominal aorta and a dissecting aneurysm distal to the renal arteries with calcification of the common iliac arteries.

Emergency surgery was done at once since rupture of the aneurysm means immediate death.

PREOPERATIVE NURSING PREPARATION

1. Practice of taking three deep breaths and then coughing.
2. Requesting medication for relief of discomfort.
3. Presence of intravenous feedings.
4. Presence of foley catheter.
5. Presence of nasogastric tube.
6. Routines and location of recovery room and surgical intensive care unit, i.e., vital signs taken frequently and visitor policies.

Since Mr. Dice's surgery was emergency in nature, as much time as was available was spent in preoperative teaching. Mr. Dice was very apprehensive when he was taken to surgery. After under anesthesia Mr. Dice's skin was prepped from the nipple line to the mid-thigh bilaterally, and a foley catheter was inserted.

OPERATIVE PROCEDURE

The operative intervention consisted of clamping the aorta and iliac arteries proximal and distal to the aneurysm for forty minutes. The aneurysm was dissected, and the lipid and calcified material removed. A dacron prosthesis was sewn proximal and distal with the aorta approximated over the prosthesis. Blood replacement was 1,000 cc. A central venous pressure catheter was inserted in the right atrium via the right antecubital vein. An arterial line was inserted into the radial artery.

Mr. Dice was taken to the recovery room while still intubated and on a MA-1 volume respirator. His condition was satisfactory.

POSTOPERATIVE NURSING CARE

1. Pulse, respirations and blood pressure every 15 min x4, then every hour
2. Morphine sulfate 8 mg I.V. every 4 hr to relieve discomfort
3. Tigan 200 mg I.M. every 4 hr for nausea
4. Central venous pressure every hour. Notify physician if over 20 mm H_2O or under 5 mm H_2O. Check with level as indicated on patient's chest. This is marked so everyone will measure from the same level.
5. Arterial blood pressure every 30 min. Notify physician if systolic over 160 mm Hg. or diastolic over 90 mm Hg.
6. Nasogastric tube to intermittent low Gomco suction
7. Hourly intake and output
8. Nothing by mouth except for few ice chips
9. MA-1 respirator set for 40% oxygen at a rate of 10 times per minute
10. Keflin 1 g intravenous every 6 hr.
11. Intravenous fluids of lactated ringers to run at 20 cc/hour plus the preceding hour's output. 500 cc low molecular dextran every 8 hr x3 days.
12. Check dorsalis pedis, posterior tibial, and popliteal pulse every hour on each leg.

POSTOPERATIVE COURSE FOR MR. DICE

Mr. Dice remained in the recovery room four hours and then was transferred to surgical intensive care (S.I.C.U.). Mr. Dice was alert on arrival to S.I.C.U. and occasionally assisted the respirator. His wife was allowed to visit him for a few minutes at this time.

Mr. Dice's vital signs stabilized. His output remained around 50–60 cc/hour. His central venous pressure remained between 6 and 8 mm water with the arterial pressure readings at 150/84 mm Hg. The first day postoperative, Mr. Dice was extubated. Mr. Dice's pulses, movement, and sensation remained excellent bilaterally. The nasogastric tube drained only a small amount of gastric juices and was removed the second day postoperative as bowel sounds had returned. Progressive ambulation was started the second day postoperative.

The third day postoperatively, Mr. Dice's central venous pressure gradually started to climb. The physician was notified. At the same time, Mr.

Dice had complained of dyspnea. An x ray showed congestion of the pulmonary veins. Mr. Dice was immediately digitalized with digoxin. The depth and rate of respirations were checked frequently. Mr. Dice was observed for other signs of congestive heart failure. There were none present. Mr. Dice's cardiac condition improved and his congestive heart failure resolved. His foley catheter was removed the fourth day postoperatively. Mr. Dice's sutures were removed the seventh day postoperatively.

DISCHARGE INSTRUCTIONS

1. No straining, pushing or pulling, i.e., heavy lifting, shoveling snow or climbing stairs or driving a car for one month.
2. Report any signs of wound drainage or increase in temperature.
3. Report any burning on urination or change in the color of the urine.
4. Report any weight gain, swelling, or edema.
5. Do not sit with legs crossed and report any pain in legs.
6. Report any pain in the abdomen.
7. Return for a clinic appointment one month later.

FOLLOW-UP VISIT

At Mr. Dice's clinic visit, he was having no complications and was allowed to return to his former job as custodian.

ADDITIONAL POINTS

Not infrequently, patients suffer paralytic ileus following this type of surgery. Therefore, some physicians suggest the use of a Miller-Abbott tube preoperatively to decompress the bowel. Also patients infrequently suffer transient paraplegia following the cross clamping of the aorta to repair the aneurysm because of interference in the blood supply to the lumbar artery supplying the spinal cord. Other complications can be incurred when the aneurysm is proximal to the renal arteries and the patient must be put on left heart bypass in order to adequately profuse the kidneys. When this occurs, you have all the extra complications that occur as the result of partial extracorporeal circulation.

STUDY GUIDE

1. Mr. Dice could have had peripheral vascular disease of arterial origin. What are the differences in peripheral vascular disease of venous and arterial origin?
2. Mr. Dice had a dissecting aneurysm. Name and describe the other two types of aortic aneurysms including the signs and symptoms they produce.
3. Mr. Dice had a Foley inserted and hourly urines ordered postoperatively.

What is the normal output per hour and why would hourly urines be important?

4. Even though Mr. Dice had emergency surgery he still had several laboratory tests performed. How would a deviation from normal in these tests affect Mr. Dice's course following surgery? List the observations for each complication the nurse could expect.

5. In abdominal aortic aneurysms why is it important for the nurse to check pulses and observe for color and temperature of the lower extremities pre- and postoperatively?

6. What complications besides those mentioned in this case could occur following surgery for an aortic aneurysm? Give the observations the nurse would make.

7. Why was Mr. Dice ambulated so early? How can the nurse determine the rate of progression for ambulation?

8. List some test results which distinguish a ruptured abdominal aneurysm from an acute myocardial infarction, acute pancreatitis, perforated peptic ulcer, and mesenteric thrombosis.

9. Distinguish between the use of a volume respirator like the MA-1 Mr. Dice was on and the pressure respirator.

10. Give some instances in which the nurse could have worked with Mr. Dice's family.

SELECTED READINGS

C. E. Anagnostopoulous, J. B. P. Manakavalan, and C. F. Kittle, "Aortic Dissections and Dissecting Aneurysms," *The American Journal of Cardiology,* August 1972, pp. 263–273.

L. S. Brunner *et al., Textbook of Medical Surgical Nursing,* 2nd ed., J. B. Lippincott, Philadelphia, 1970.

P. B. Buson and W. McDermott, *Cecil-Loeb Textbook of Medicine,* W. B. Saunders, Philadelphia, 1971.

B. Chow, "Aortic Aneurysm—A Patient Study," *Nursing Clinics of North America,* March 1969, pp. 131–141.

M. Delp and R. Manning, *Major's Physical Diagnosis,* 7th ed., W. B. Saunders, Philadelphia, 1968.

L. S. Goodman and A. Gilman, *Pharmacological Basis of Therapeutics,* 4th ed., Macmillan, London, 1970.

P. L. daLuz, "Congestive Heart Failure Following Abdominal Surgery," *Heart and Lung,* vol. 1, no. 6, November–December 1972, pp. 835–839.

J. McFarland *et al.,* "The Medical Treatment of Dissecting Aortic Aneurysms," *The New England Journal of Medicine,* January 20, 1972, pp. 115–120.

Mr. John Archer

seventy-five years old

Right Hemiplegia/ Acute Chronic

Lily Larson

Mr. John Archer, age seventy-five, lives in a lower middle-class neighborhood with his wife, Ella. They have three married sons who are all living in different parts of the United States, the closest living about 150 miles from Mr. and Mrs. Archer. Mr. Archer has been a house painter all his life, he owns his own two-story home which is old but well kept. Mr. Archer, although past retirement, has worked consistently at his trade, but slowed down since the development of bilateral cataracts. He had them removed about six months before his "stroke." His wife said he was able to see well enough to read and to "get around," but had some trouble adjusting to stairways.

The following was revealed to the visiting nurse several weeks after his hospitalization. "When I woke up, my whole right side was paralyzed. I had no feeling in it at all. I tried to get out of bed, but couldn't make it. I tried to figure out what happened to me, but couldn't remember. I didn't have any more to drink than usual—a few beers and a highball at bedtime." (He began to consume alcoholic beverages when the cataracts were impairing his ability to work.) "I was a bit frightened. My wife called the doctor, and he sent me to the hospital in an ambulance. I can't remember arriving at the hospital."

ADMISSION NOTE

Sunday A.M., Mr. Archer was admitted via stretcher ambulance, semiconscious and in some respiratory distress. 9 A.M.: Oxygen was administered per mask; blood pressure 200/110; pulse 86; respiration 22; temperature 37.8°C rectally; respiration stertorous; face flushed; pupils dilated, react to light.

PHYSICAL EXAM

Mr. Archer was semiconscious, confused and disoriented during the physical exam. He did not respond verbally to questions. Mrs. Archer was the historian.

230

Past medical history: No significant illness until this year in which he had bilateral senile cataracts which were removed successfully. Right cataract removed in January 1972, and left in February 1972.

Nocturia: 2–3 times nightly.

Eyes: Clear; pupils respond to light; dilated; corneal reflexes present; aphakic.

Movements: Unable to test.

Ears: Drums intact; no history of impairment of hearing.

Nose: Clear; septum deviates to left.

Mouth: Edentulous, wears dentures; tongue deviates slightly to left.

Abdomen: Negative.

Extremities: Flaccid right side (arm and leg); questionable response to pin prick, right side; responds to pain, left side; Babinski on right side.

Impression: Cerebral thrombosis, left middle cerebral artery; paralysis right side with questionable aphasia.

Rule out: Aneurysm.

Problems: Benign prostatic hypertrophy, nocturia, shortness of breath.

MEDICAL ORDERS

1. Oxygen, nasal catheter: 6–8 liters per min.
2. Suction p.r.n.
3. Foley catheter #16 F. with 5 cc bag.
4. Serpasil (reserpine) 0.5 mg I.M. q. 4 h. for systolic B.P. above 180 mm.
5. A.S.A. 500 mg rectally q. 4–6 h. for temp. above 38.5° (R).
6. Chloral hydrate 0.5 g rectal suppository q. 6 h., p.r.n. for restlessness.
7. Check response to verbal and pain stimuli q.h.
8. Lumbar puncture, stat.
9. B.P., P., and resp. q. 30 min. q. 4 h. thereafter q.h. until stable.
10. Lab: U.A., C.B.C., prothrombin time, cholesterol, electrolytes, and CO_2 combining power in A.M.
11. 1,500 cc 5% dextrose distilled water with one Amp. B Complex and Vit. C, I.V. stat, for 24 hr.
12. Clear liquids when tolerated.
13. I&O.
14. ECG today.

ACTIONS OF NURSE

Carried out medical orders and carried out the following:

1. Inserted nasal catheter, continuous oxygen—7 liters per minute. Supervised attendant in inserting Foley catheter to dependent drainage.
2. 10 A.M., prepared intravenous infusion and set drop rate at 20 drops per minute.
3. Oro-pharyngeal suctioning to stimulate coughing and remove secretions.
4. Mouth care: 3x daily; inserted dentures which his wife brought.
5. Back massage at 12, 3, and 9 P.M.

Body alignment: Trochanter roll to right hip when in supine position; elevation of head—35° angle; pillow under right arm; extend fingers over roll; foot board.

6. Reposition every 3 hr.
7. Side rails.
8. Check for level of consciousness.
9. Passive full range of motion of all joints twice daily.
10. Observe intravenous drop rate.
11. Vital signs as prescribed.
12. Record intake and output.

P.M. DAY OF ADMISSION

Observations: Eyes half open; ptosis of right eyelid; right cheek more flaccid than left. Eye movements upon verbal stimulation; pupils respond to light. Right hand is limp; flexed on chest; hand closed. Some grasp in left hand. Right leg flexed and externally rotated; foot in plantar flexion. As nurse adjusts pillow, neck appears pulled toward left. Mr. Archer responds with a grunt to stimuli. Does not answer questions. Results of spinal puncture is essentially negative. Pressure slightly increased.

9 P.M.: Intake 10 A.M.–9 P.M. 700 cc; output 550 cc.

FIRST HOSPITAL DAY—A.M. OBSERVATIONS

Vital signs: blood pressure dropping slowly. 11 A.M., 180/90; 12 noon, 175/90; 1 P.M., 170/86.

Checked laboratory reports: complete blood count: hemoglobin 9 grams, hematocrit 30%, white blood count 15,000.

Differential: lymphocytes 59, monocytes 2, eosinophiles 0 basophiles 0.

Prothrombin 13 seconds or 85%, 12 seconds control

Sodium—140 milliequivalents
Chlorides—100 milliequivalents
Potassium—4 milliequivalents

Serum cholesterol—295 mg/100 cc serum

Blood urea nitrogen—16 mg/100 cc

Urinalysis: specific gravity 1.03; pH 5; albumin 3+

6 P.M.—blood pressure 170/90, pulse 78, temperature by rectum 38.2°C

7 P.M.—restlessness
   Chloral hydrate rectal suppository .5 g
   Sips of water—no dysphagia

24 hr intake 1,580 cc, output 1,350 cc
   Intravenous is patent
   No respiratory distress
   Vital signs stable
   Chloral hydrate repeated at 2 A.M.
   Position changed every 3 hr during night
   Observations by night nurse: Slept at hour intervals (approximately 4 hr).

7 A.M.—NURSE'S ACTIONS

Nurse read chart.

As she approached Mr. Archer and touched his left hand, she said, "good morning." His response was a squeeze of her hand and an attempt to talk.

He moved his lips, but no sound emitted.
   Nurse: "Mr. Archer, do you know that you are in the hospital?"
   He nodded.
   "You came in yesterday. Do you remember what happened?"
   Mr. Archer nodded his head as he looked at the nurse.

Conversations by nurse—
   Nurse: "Dr. Jackson talked with you last night, did he not?"
   Patient: Did not respond verbally, but shook his head.
   Nurse: "Do you know why you came to the hospital?"
   Patient: Pointed to right leg and arm.
   Nurse: "You had a stroke and you're in the hospital where we can help you."
   Patient: Nodded.
   Nurse: "The doctor explained to your wife what happened and about your medical treatment?"
   Patient: Shook head.
   Nurse: "Your wife called and said that her neighbor was bringing her to

see you this morning. She will be bringing your eye glasses. Can you see me?"

Patient: Nodded, "yes."

Nurse: "In the meantime, we have some work to do to make you feel better."

Bath, back care, nose care, mouth care, catheter care given. Position changed.

Vital signs stable. Urine clear, adequate.

8:30 A.M.—Tea and ginger ale tolerated well; some drooling, right side.

9:30 A.M.—Dr. Jackson visited.

NEW MEDICAL ORDERS

Discontinue O_2.

Full liquid diet as tolerated.

Continued with infusions: 5,000 units heparin per 1,000 cc of 5% dextrose in distilled water for next 24 hr.

Type-cross-match for 1 unit of blood.

Clotting time.

Vital signs every 4 hr.

Findings: Electrocardiogram report, sinus rhythm and rate normal; tracings suggest mild ventricular hypertrophy.

Mrs. Archer arrived in time to talk with the physician. Dr. Jackson told Mrs. Archer that Mr. Archer is in good physical health except for the stroke and anemia. Mrs. Archer asked if Mr. Archer could have a highball at night as he was accustomed to having several at bedtime for the past several months. Dr. Jackson told the nurse that Mr. Archer could have one ounce of alcoholic beverage as tolerated at bedtime. Mrs. Archer would bring a bottle of bourbon to the hospital. The nurse wrote this on the physician's order sheet as a verbal order which Dr. Jackson later signed.

As Mrs. Archer entered the room accompanied by the nurse, Mr. Archer reached out his hand to his wife and started to cry. Mr. Archer pointed to his mouth. Mrs. Archer said, "I know, John," as she held his hand, "but they say that you will be well again and able to talk." The nurse, as she left the room, informed Mr. Archer to use the call light (which she placed near his left hand) if they needed her.

NURSE'S OBSERVATIONS AND ACTIONS

12:30 P.M.
Mr. Archer drank ½ glass of milk, beef broth, and ate the custard. Position changed. Mouth care given.

3:00 P.M.
Mr. Archer's neighbor (Mr. Dorn, about fifty-five years of age) arrived. Mrs. Archer talked with him before entering the room. He stayed for twenty minutes. Mrs. Archer left with Mr. Dorn and said that she would be back in the evening.

3:30 P.M.
Mr. Archer's position changed.
Infusion running.

5:00 P.M.
Mr. Archer has slept for 1½ hours.

6:30 P.M.
Physician visited. Noted oral intake of 500 cc since 7 A.M.

MEDICAL ORDERS

Discontinue intravenous after completed.
Warfarin sodium 5 mg by mouth in the A.M.
Prothrombin time daily.

7:30 P.M.
Mrs. Archer visiting.
Nurse raised head of bed after asking Mr. Archer if he wished to sit up straighter.

9:00 P.M.
12 hr intake: 1,800 cc; output: 1,550 cc.
Back care; turned; dentures cleaned; mouth care given.
Extremities placed and supported in alignment.
Given 1 oz whisky in 100 cc ginger ale.

Mr. Archer has been repositioned every 2–3 hr. Slept most of the night.

SECOND HOSPITAL DAY

Blood started at 30 gtts./min. Vital signs stable. Taking fluids well.

8:00 A.M.
Back care given; elevated head of bed; placed over-bed table in front of Mr. Archer. Mr. Archer picked up his glasses with his left hand and the

nurse assisted him in placing them. He smiled. The nurse noted some drooping of the right side of his face. The nurse decided to encourage Mr. Archer to help with his morning care. First, however, she wanted to know how well he could identify articles. She then placed a glass of water, a comb, a tooth brush, and a wash cloth on the stand. As the nurse called out the articles, Mr. Archer pointed to each one after some groping. The nurse then asked Mr. Archer to close his eyes and touch his right arm with his left hand, which he did.

"That's fine. I just wanted to make sure that you understood me when I talked with you."

The nurse then explained why she wanted Mr. Archer to take several deep breaths every few hours and demonstrated deep-breathing to the patient.

She also explained and showed Mr. Archer how to move his left arm and leg through range of motion. He immediately followed her direction.

The nurse described the results of the tests she had done on Mr. Archer's record, which the physician read.

10:00 A.M.
Dr. Jackson and Miss Lee, the nurse, visited Mr. Archer. Dr. Jackson informed the patient that he was doing very well and that the blood would help him feel stronger. He also told Mr. Archer that they would soon begin exercises and speech practice. "The sooner we start, the easier it will be for you to strengthen your right side and to relearn the use of your mouth in talking." Later to Miss Lee, Dr. Jackson said, "It is quite early to begin rehabilitation, but if all goes well today, I think we will have physical therapy and speech therapy started tomorrow."

MEDICAL ORDERS

Soft diet as tolerated.

12:30 P.M.
Miss Lee noted that Mr. Archer's drooling had nearly subsided. Fed self with assistance. After dinner, Mr. Archer appeared tired. After changing Mr. Archer's position and giving him a backrub, Miss Lee noted that he fell asleep. Miss Lee met Mrs. Archer at the nurses' station, explaining to Mrs. Archer that Mr. Archer was having a transfusion to give him more energy. Since Mr. Archer was sleeping, Mrs. Archer remained in the visitors' lounge at the suggestion of Miss Lee. Miss Lee sat down with Mrs. Archer for two reasons: to establish rapport with her and to learn more about Mr. and Mrs. Archer's activities, habits, and diet. The nurse also was able to assess Mrs. Archer's understanding of Mr. Archer's illness. Miss Lee indicated to Mrs. Archer that she would be available for

questions and assistance to both Mr. and Mrs. Archer. The nurse decided that she should tell Mrs. Archer that her husband might become discouraged and blue at times during recovery and rehabilitation and that her encouragement would be very important. Mrs. Archer told the nurse she had a neighbor who had a stroke who has never gotten out of bed, but can read and speak. "Do you think my husband will be this way?" The nurse responded, "It is a little early to know, but we are encouraged with his progress. The doctor is already planning physical and speech therapy."

Miss Lee obtained the following information from Mrs. Archer:

Rest and sleep pattern: 8–10 hours, drinks beer and bourbon before going to bed. Naps some in afternoon.

Breathing: No shortness of breath until stroke. Does not smoke.

Fluids: Beer, milk, highball at bedtime.

Eating: Meat and potatoes. Bread and milk. Does not eat much fruit or vegetables.

Elimination: Takes milk of magnesia 2–3 times a week and magnesium sulfate when no results from milk of magnesia. Expects bowels to move daily. Constipated frequently.

Bladder: Nocturia 2 times last several months.

Significant others: Wife; two neighbors, same age group as the Archers; grown children visit occasionally.

Wife's understanding of disease: Needs to be informed of changes. She is apprehensive and intelligent. She wants to be involved in husband's care.

THIRD HOSPITAL DAY

Actions of Nurse

Mr. Archer reached for the alphabet cards and spelled out, "No toilet," and pointed to his abdomen. The alphabet cards had been obtained by the nurse from occupational therapy. The nurse palpated his abdomen and noted that it was soft and asked, "Are you uncomfortable?" Mr. Archer shook his head and with effort said "no." Miss Lee: "How often do you usually have a bowel movement?"

Mr. Archer pointed to two fingers. Miss Lee explained that he hasn't had much activity, and he probably would not have them as regularly as before because of his limited activity. She said however that she would call Dr. Jackson's attention to this matter.

Taking fluids satisfactorily. Passive range of motion. Noted some spasticity of right leg.

MEDICAL ORDERS

Dulcolax suppository
Vital signs, b.i.d.
Diet as tolerated
Remove Foley catheter
Consultation with speech therapist
Consultation with physical therapist

Actions of Nurse

Removed Foley catheter, continued monitoring intake and output.

Wrote on Kardex, "Force fluids; offer urinal every 4 hr; has nocturia."

During the afternoon, the nurse observed Mr. Archer crying. When asked if something was wrong, he shook his head "no" and turned his face away from the nurse. Nurse left Mr. Archer at this time and came back half an hour later.

FOURTH HOSPITAL DAY

The physical therapist visited Mr. Archer. Miss Lee chose to remain with the patient. The physical therapist gave range of motion to all extremities and explained the reasons to the patient. She showed how he could go through range of motion using his non-paralyzed extremities.

During the speech therapist's visit, the nurse chose not to stay in the room. Speech therapist findings: Motor aphasia with moderate apraxia. (Patient able to blow out flame of match, but with difficulty.) Can say simple words such as "yes" or "no." Plans: Will begin practicing with vowels. Will need to relearn each sound used in speech. Will increase to one syllable words, then two, etc. Mr. Archer seems well motivated.

The nurse noted that Mr. Archer's temperature was 38.4°C and reported this to the doctor who said the elevation was likely due to cystitis and ordered a culture and sensitivity as well as a complete urinalysis.

Mr. Archer was exhausted by 3:30 P.M. and slept at short intervals during the afternoon. The nurse increased his fluid intake. Mrs. Archer was apprised of his need to take fluids.

FIFTH HOSPITAL DAY

Medical orders:
Sulfisoxazole 1 g stat and then 500 mg q. 4 h.
Force fluids.

Mr. Archer went to physical therapy once today; speech therapy once.

SIXTH HOSPITAL DAY

Encouraged to bathe more of self (use of sponge rather than wash cloth).
Medical orders:
To have carotid angiogram in A.M. Long support-hose.
Demerol 50 mg I.M. on call
Atropine .6 mg I.M. on call

Post angiogram orders:
Ice pack to left neck for 2 hours.
Darvon 65 mg P.O. every 4 hr p.r.n. for pain.
Cancel physical therapy for tomorrow.
Resume other pre-angiogram orders 4 hr after angiogram if no complications.

SEVENTH HOSPITAL DAY

Report of angiogram: 2% Xylocaine injected. 25 cc of 50% Hypaque (radio-opaque) solution injected into left common carotid artery. Normal carotid distention. Films of neck, frontal and lateral exposures were made serially. Normal delineation of the internal carotid artery and its major branches. No displacement of structure.

EIGHTH TO THIRTEENTH HOSPITAL DAYS

Mr. Archer continued to progress.

THIRTEENTH HOSPITAL DAY

Nurse assisted patient to wheelchair to physical therapy.
Speech therapy: Mr. Archer is able to say many one-syllable words intelligibly; however, he is unable to say words that begin with the letters P and F.

SIXTEENTH HOSPITAL DAY

Mr. Archer is able to put some weight on right leg for the first time. Patient to physical therapy in wheelchair.

When Mr. Archer returned from physical therapy, he said, "Good to out room." The nurse said, "You are speaking very well, Mr. Archer, but you leave out some words. Try to say a full sentence." Mr. Archer replied, "No good for anything. Gettin' too old." The nurse patted him and said, "You're not too old, John. You're in fine health except for your muscle weakness, and you're getting stronger. Today you did put some weight on your leg for the first time. That's a good sign." Mr. Archer turned away with tears in his eyes.

Nurse: "I'm sure you're discouraged because you're not as active as you used to be, but we'll work together on those muscles."

POST-HOSPITALIZATION

Public health nurse, referral: Visit to home just previous to dismissal. Recommended: Scatter rugs be removed and a wood stool or chair be placed in the bathtub over the rubber suction mats which were already in the tub. Helped Mrs. Archer obtain a wheelchair and a commode. Nurse assessed Mrs. Archer's knowledge of Mr. Archer's nutritional needs. Mrs. Archer expressed concern about Mr. Archer wanting to return to drinking four highballs each evening and that she didn't see how they could afford this. The nurse recommended substituting hot chocolate since Mr. Archer had drunk this frequently while in the hospital, and said that she would return soon after Mr. Archer's dismissal from the hospital to see if they needed anything.

SUMMARY—REHABILITATION PROGRAM

In spite of frequent frustration and periods of depression, Mr. Archer was discharged to his home where arrangements had been made for physical therapy and public health nursing assistance. A neighbor planned to visit (and did) during the day and along with Mrs. Archer was taught how to assist Mr. Archer when he was moving from bed to chair and from a chair to a standing position.

Initially after dismissal from the hospital, the neighbor and Mrs. Archer tended to do things for Mr. Archer that he could do for himself. However, with guidance from the public health nurse, Mrs. Archer began encouraging Mr. Archer and he resumed his rehabilitation schedule. Mrs. Archer told the nurse that, at times, she felt sorry for her husband who often became discouraged when progress was slow. The public health nurse observed that Mr. Archer refused to feed himself and was reluctant to carry out his rehabilitation schedule at times. He also became more demanding of his wife's attentions. Mrs. Archer had been reluctant to allow visitors previous to this time, and Mr. Archer was opposed to having visitors because he didn't want people to see "how he was." The nurse suggested that they invite a few of their close friends to visit occasionally. Following this, Mr. and Mrs. Archer began attending church again.

One of Mr. Archer's friends, who is also a house painter, asked Mr. Archer to paint an unfinished bird house, which Mr. Archer enjoyed doing very much.

Within six months after returning home, the nurse reported that Mr. Archer was speaking well, but with some hesitation, and he was walking with the aid of a cane. He experienced weakness in his right arm only when becoming tired. Mr. Archer was dismissed from the public health agency seven months after hospital dismissal. At this time, he had achieved essential return to the level of activity that he had previous to the CVA, with moderation in activity typical of retirement.

SPEECH AND LANGUAGE PROCESS

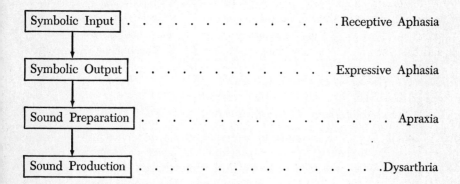

Symbolic Input	. . . . Receptive Aphasia
Symbolic Output	. . . . Expressive Aphasia
Sound Preparation	. . . . Apraxia
Sound Production	. . . . .Dysarthria

DEFINITIONS

Speech: Any sound that can be produced in the vocal tract. In English, these sounds are either vowels or consonants.

Language: A system of symbols that communicates ideas.

Aphasia: Inability to voluntarily initiate speech movements. Chewing and swallowing functions are intact.

Dysarthria: Inability to voluntarily initiate movements of oral musculature. Chewing and swallowing are affected.

LANGUAGE INVENTORY FOR NURSING STAFF

WORKING WITH——————————————— FLOOR————

1. Does the patient have difficulty in chewing and swallowing?
   yes———— no————
2. The patient expresses his/her needs, a/ by asking ( ), b/ by using gestures ( ), c/ does not talk ( ). CHECK.
3. The patient speaks, a/ in sentences ( ), b/ in single words ( ), c/ does not talk ( ). CHECK.
4. Does the patient appear to understand when *you* speak to him?
   yes———— no————

5. When the patient speaks, are you able to understand the words?
   yes————— no—————
6. Does the patient appear frustrated if he is unable to make himself understood? yes————— no—————
7. Is the patient ambulatory? yes————— no—————
8. Is the patient near a T.V. or a radio? yes————— no—————
   Does the patient appear to understand when watching and/or listening?
   yes————— no—————
9. Please list some of the things the patient needs to ask for in the hospital:
10. Other remarks:

HOW THE NURSE AND OTHER HOSPITAL STAFF CONCERNED WITH THE CASE OF AN APHASIC PATIENT CAN HELP WITH THE REHABILITATION OF THE PATIENT'S SPEECH

1. Anticipating what the patient is trying to say by voicing it for him, markedly impedes progress in speech and language development. Always encourage the patient to speak and do for himself, but never make *an issue* over his doing it. If he can read, encourage him to read the newspaper; if he can write his name, encourage him to sign his name rather than make a cross for his signature. Let him take care of his grooming and his physical needs as much as possible.

2. Accept an aphasic patient *as he is.* Let him express himself freely on his own speech and language level. Exert every effort to understand what he is trying to tell you whether it be in words, distorted syllables, or pantomime.

3. If the patient swears, or voices emotional utterances, *avoid any show of disapproval.* To express annoyance or reprove a patient only inhibits his attempts at communication and may cause withdrawal "into his shell."

4. Avoid putting pressure on a patient to get him to utter a complete sentence. If he says only the essential words (e.g., nouns, pronouns, and action verbs), show pleasure over such speech efforts. Brief utterances made during early post-traumatic days are most acceptable efforts, and they should be praised.

5. When handing the patient an object such as a fork, repeat the word "fork" several times. Say it in a confident, modulated voice—never a rising, questioning inflection. Similarly, when bathing any part of the patient's body, say the name of that part several times as you wash it. At first, arm, hand, leg, foot, toe, etc. Later, use such words as back, ear, face, chin, etc. Use only one-syllable words at first, then two-syllable words such as shoulder, elbow, etc.

6. Should the patient indicate a desire to be helped with a word, pronounce

it slowly and distinctly. Avoid saying, "Watch me as I say it," or "Put your tongue here or there," or the like. Directions regarding correct use of speech musculature are handled by the speech pathologist during therapy sessions. Most speech pathologists will discuss and demonstrate to the attendant what can be done to help the patient, especially if he requests such assistance.

7. Avoid saying, "Now relax, and then you say it." To tell the aphasic to relax is distracting and upsetting. You may even precipitate an anxiety attack. Assume a calm, friendly attitude and avoid any show of concern or anxiety when he has difficulty in responding.

Courtesy of the Department of Speech and Hearing, University of Kansas Medical Center.

STUDY GUIDE

1. "Prevention" or delay of impending strokes are more recent concepts. What is the profile of people who are potentially considered high risk?
2. What are the health measures health personnel should teach in prevention or delay?
3. What are the warning signs and symptoms of stroke?
4. Describe the pathophysiology of Mr. Archer's stroke.
5. What are the nursing observations and assessments during the acute stage of Mr. Archer's stroke—the period of time he may be semiconscious, unconscious, or comatose?
6. Should Mr. Archer's temperature rise suddenly to 39–40°C early in his hospitalization, what might this indicate?
7. What are the nursing goals and actions during the acute stage regarding:
   a. Oxygenation
   b. Body alignment
   c. Fluid requirement
   d. Urinary problems
8. If the spinal fluid were bloody, what might be the type of cerebral damage? Prognosis?
9. How would you respond to Mrs. Archer when she says, "I wonder if he'll be like one of our friends who just lays there and never talks."
10. Discuss the rationale for administering heparin, coumadin.
11. Why is it necessary to check prothrombin time?
12. What are nursing observations necessary during heparinization? Why?
13. What directions would you give a patient who is on anticoagulant therapy at home?
14. After Mr. Archer is aware of his environment, plan care regarding:
    a. Bladder training
    b. Feeding

15. How would you determine whether or not Mr. Archer has homonomous hemanopsia? How does a nurse help a patient who has this kind of pathology?
16. Why did the nurse place articles in front of Mr. Archer and ask him to identify them?
17. How do you help the patient do his own passive range of motion on the paralyzed side?
18. Mr. Archer has motor aphasia. How can the nurse help Mr. Archer to relearn to talk?
19. Mr. Archer has a good potential for rehabilitation. What, in Mr. Archer's case, would be your actions in helping Mr. and Mrs. Archer reach his maximum potential of functioning?

SELECTED READINGS

A. S. Abramson and E. F. Delagi, "Influence of Weight Bearing and Muscle Contraction on Disuse Osteoporosis," *Archives of Physical Medicine and Rehabilitation,* vol. 46, March 1965, pp. 147–151.

M. Adams, M. Baron, and M. A. Caston, "Urinary Incontinence in the Acute Phase or Cerebral Vascular Accident," *Nursing Research,* vol. 15, Spring 1966, pp. 100–108. (Good review of literature.)

I. Beland, *Clinical Nursing,* Macmillan, New York, 1965, pp. 1240–1273.

Daniel R. Boone, *An Adult Has Aphasia,* Interstate Printers and Publishers, Danville, Ill., 1965.

L. S. Brunner, L. P. Emerson *et al., Textbook of Medical-Surgical Nursing,* 2nd ed., J. B. Lippincott, Philadelphia, 1971, pp. 792–798.

M. W. Buck, "Adjustments During Recovery from Stroke," *American Journal of Nursing,* vol. 64, no. 10, October 1964, pp. 92–95.

C. G. De Gutierrez-Mahoney and E. Carine, *Neurological and Neurosurgical Nursing,* 4th ed., C. V. Mosby, St. Louis, 1965, pp. 42–48, 53–57, 64–70, 252–261, 297–298.

Sister Regina Elizabeth, "Sensory Stimulation Techniques," *American Journal of Nursing,* vol. 66, February 1966, pp. 281–286.

William Fields, *Pathogenesis and Treatment of Cerebrovascular Disease,* Charles Thomas, Springfield, Ill., 1961, pp. 222–237.

William S. Fields and William A. Spencer, *Stroke Rehabilitation: Basic Concepts and Research Trends,* Warren H. Green, St. Louis, 1967.

Alvin I. Goldfarb, "Responsibilities to Our Aged," *American Journal of Nursing,* vol. 64, no. 11, November 1964, pp. 77–83.

Margaret A. Goode, "The Patient with a Cerebral Vascular Accident," *Nursing Outlook,* vol. 14, no. 3, March 1966, pp. 60–62.

Eric Hodgins, *Episode: Report on the Accident Inside My Skull,* Atheneum, New York, 1964.

Irene Hullicka, "Fostering Self-Respect in Aged Patients," *American Journal of Nursing*, vol. 64, no. 3, March 1964, pp. 84–89.

Mieczyslaw Pesczynki, "The Rehabilitation Potential of the Late Adult Hemiplegic," *American Journal of Nursing*, vol. 63, no. 4, April 1963, pp. 111–114.

B. K. Piskor and S. Paleos, "The Group Way to Banish After-Stroke Blues," *American Journal of Nursing*, vol. 68, no. 7, July 1968, pp. 1500–1503.

Irene Ramey, "The Stroke Patient is Interesting," *Nursing Forum*, vol. 6, no. 3, pp. 67, 273–279.

Robert Sautell and G. M. Martin, "Perceptual Problems of the Hemiplegic Patient," *The Journal Lancet*, vol. 87, June 1967, pp. 193–196.

Herbert A. Schoening and Frederic J. Kottke, "Rehabilitation of the Patient with Hemi-plegia," *Current Therapy*, W. B. Saunders, Philadelphia, 1966, p. 561.

Lucie Schultz, *The Stroke Patient.* Paper presented at the American Heart Association meeting, Council of C.V. Nursing, Dallas, Texas, November 1969.

Kathryn M. Suggs, "Coping and Adaptive Behavior in the Stroke Syndrome," *Nursing Forum*, no. 1, 1971, pp. 100–111.

James Taren, "Cerebral Aneurysm," *American Journal of Nursing*, vol. 65, no. 4, April 1965, pp. 88–95.

Montaque Ullman, "Disorders of Body Image after Stroke," *American Journal of Nursing*, vol. 64, no. 10, October 1964, pp. 89–91.

Frederick A. Whitehouse, "Stroke: The Present Challenge," *Nursing Forum*, no. 1, 1971, pp. 90–91.

PAMPHLETS

American Heart Association. *Do It Yourself Again.* New York: American Heart Association, 1965.

American Heart Association. *Up and Around.* New York: American Heart Association, 1965.

Kenny Rehabilitation Institute. *Rehabilitative Nursing Techniques.* Minneapolis, Minnesota: Kenny Rehabilitation, 1962–1964.
1. Bed Positioning and Transfer Procedures for the Hemiplegic.
2. Selected Equipment Useful in the Hospital, Home, or Nursing Home.
3. A Procedure for Passive Range of Motion and Self-Assistive Exercises.
4. Self-Care and Homemaking for the Hemiplegic.